CORE TRUTHS

Empowering Women to Understand and Change Core Muscles for Optimal Health

Dr. Luci Bennett, PT, DPT

This book is not intended as a substitute for the medical advice of physicians. The reader should consult a physician in matters relating to her health and particularly with respect to any symptoms that may require diagnosis or medical attention.

ISBN: 978-1-7326475-6-5
Ebook ISBN: 978-1-7326475-7-2

Image licensing granted by SciePro, Chu KyungMin, Shutterstock.com

Edited by Jennifer Holder
https://fullbloompublications.com

Cover and interior layout by Mayfly Design
https://mayflydesign.com

Interior photography by Therapy Illustrated LLC
Author photo by Thomas Faulkenberry

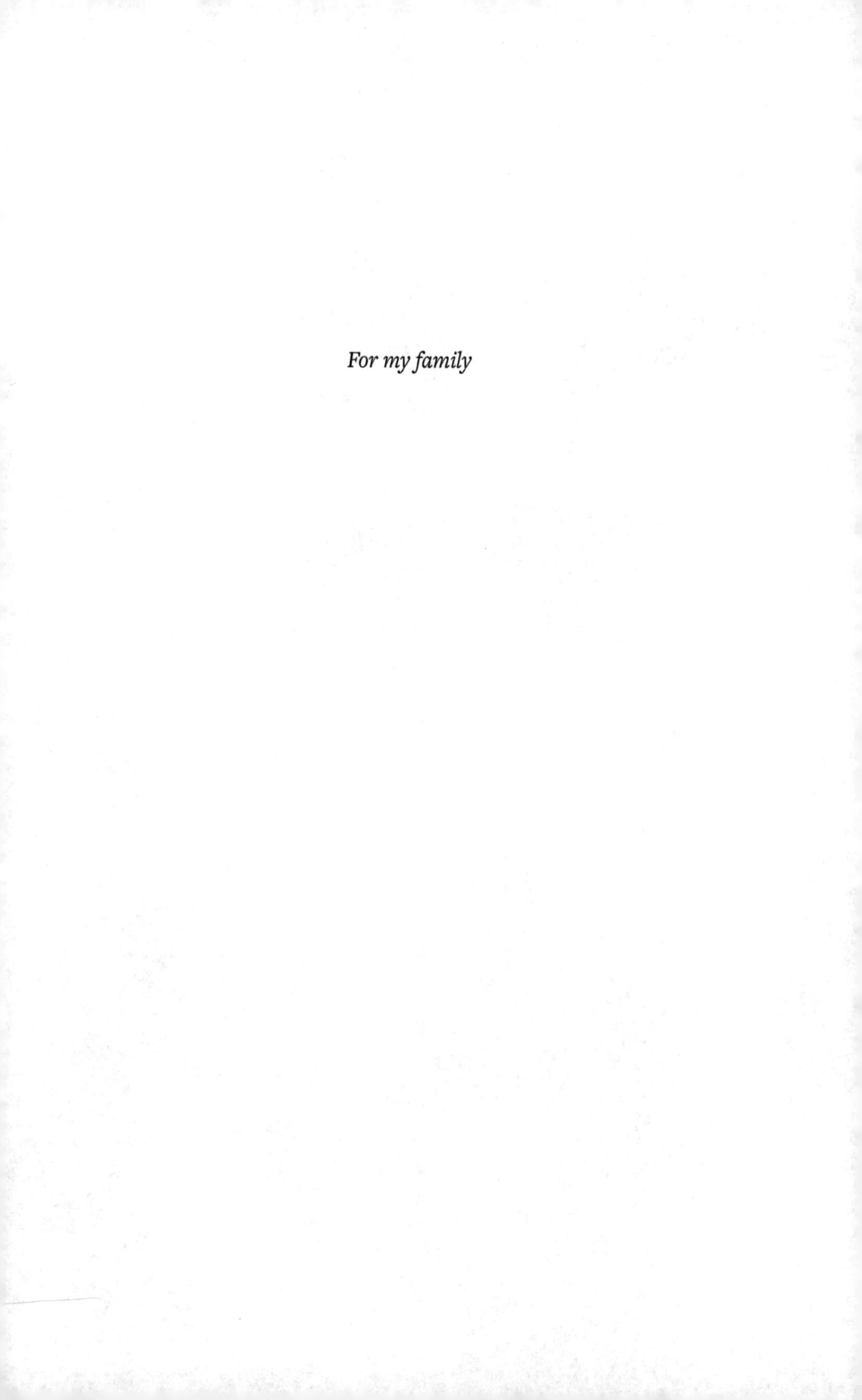

For my family

Contents

Introduction: Prioritize Your Body's Unique Needs vii

Part One: Understand Just What You Are Doing

CHAPTER 1: The Science Beyond Fads and Internet Advice 3

CHAPTER 2: Anatomy of Core Muscles 17

CHAPTER 3: Essentials of Pressure Mechanics 29

CHAPTER 4: Truths About Core Strength and Core Control 39

Part Two: Core Struggles and the Painful Consequences

CHAPTER 5: Musculoskeletal Pain 51

CHAPTER 6: Organ Consequences 61

CHAPTER 7: Pregnancy 69

CHAPTER 8: Incontinence and Pelvic Organ Prolapse 79

CHAPTER 9: Asthma and Chronic Obstructive Pulmonary Disease ... 89

CHAPTER 10: Functional Gastrointestinal Disorders 99

CHAPTER 11: Back Pain 105

CHAPTER 12: Osteoporosis 115

Part Three: Restore Your Inner Core

CHAPTER 13: Evaluate Your Core 125

CHAPTER 14: Core Focus Exercises 139

CHAPTER 15: Core Gravity Exercises 147

CHAPTER 16: Core Function Exercises 163

CHAPTER 17: Integrating the Core 169

Conclusion: Core Grace for Moving Forward 177

References 183

INTRODUCTION

Prioritize Your Body's Unique Needs

There may be a lot of reasons why you have decided to embrace a change and are motivated to strengthen your core. Perhaps it's because you want to improve the way you look and flatten down that belly. Maybe it's because you have a nagging, persistent pain somewhere in your back. There are many women with many different stories and motivations. You could be like Sara, Rita, or Helen—or you may be like all of them.

Sara loves baking cakes for special events. But she can barely assume the decorating position: gripping the angle of the piping bag, eyes aligning its tip to the cake, in a slightly stooped posture. Sara can hardly last minutes in this stance before her back muscles give out and freeze up in pain. She grits her teeth and rushes the swirl before dropping the bag of icing to clutch her back. None of her cakes turn out right anymore, mostly because she is in pain before she can finish.

When Rita arrives at a Pictionary party and sees that Hadi is there, she immediately wishes she hadn't worn khaki pants. Hadi always cracks jokes that send the entire room into hysterics. Though Rita loves a good laugh, she knows it will make her pee her pants. If only she had worn black! If only she weren't too embarrassed to ask her host for a pad! Then she could have a good time without worry and shame. Rita thinks incontinence is just something you have to live with.

Helen avoided getting fitted for her bridesmaid dress for as long as her sister could tolerate it. Even though Helen is only in her early forties, she looks more and more like a much older woman with a very rounded back and a large pooch in her belly. She has been suffering from a flare-up of irritable bowel syndrome (IBS) for over a month; plus, she just met with a surgeon to fix her prolapse. She feels miserable more often than not. Every day, she tries to get through the core exercises that others make look so easy, but she swears they are making her feel worse. Helen can't lose weight no matter how little she eats. It is true, the mirror is not Helen's friend, and none of the bridesmaid dresses work out. While the tailor comes up with an alternative cut for her dress, Helen goes home despondent. She is losing hope for her body.

If you have sought help for challenges like these from physicians, physical therapists, fitness coaches, or trainers, they will all educate you by saying that a strong core is important for a healthy back. They also say that a strong core is important for balance. These are core truths.

But the primary truth of core exercise is that successful training of the core is complex—getting the results you want is not as simple as a "Top Twenty Core Exercises" program. This is particularly true for women—and it has nothing to do with being the "weaker sex"! Training a woman's core requires understanding how the business works. Core muscles do a whole lot more than crunch, plank, and lift heavy weights.

To put it simply, women's bodies are different than men's bodies, and achieving core health is much tougher for us. We experience constant changes and hormonal fluctuations that affect our body's chemistry. Men do not have these challenges, aches, and pains on a monthly basis. A woman's body may not respond to core exercise the same way a man's will, especially as we age. A high percentage of women develop more significant painful side effects to these "Top Twenty" exercises—side effects and problems that men rarely, if ever, have to contend with.

Don't get me wrong: Men and women certainly share the same set of muscles and bones, but there are differences. These are differences I like to call "Lady Business" because the physiological business of being a lady is simply different than a man's physiology. Lady Business includes things like estrogen and testosterone, which can strongly affect the connective tissue and stability of bone. We have an extra organ men don't have—the uterus. We have a different configuration to our bottoms. We have babies. It is this collection of anatomical and physiological differences, or Lady Business, along with many other changes in our bodies that happen with life, that can set women up for core troubles.

Core Troubles Women Experience

The most obvious trouble that people run into is pain: pain in the low back, pain in the upper back, pain in the neck, pain of the pelvis. These are a few choice examples. Pain associated with the spine and pelvis is a muscle problem. Core problems are muscle problems. When core muscles are not doing their job of holding the bones and controlling how the bones move, then inflammation sets in and we experience pain.

There are other jobs that core muscles are responsible for, and if the core isn't working well, then there is trouble. This set of muscles also has to breathe, support the organ system, manage the internal pressures, and hold continence. These are not the first things we think of when considering core muscles. In fact, most people believe the core is just the Six-Pack muscle. But there is much more to it.

How the Diaphragm is working is critical to how the entire core performs. Although most people do not associate breath with core exercise and the Diaphragm with core muscles, they are essential for supporting the base of the rib cage with the spine, as well as for reinforcing the muscles by pressurizing the internal pressure system. Everybody has resorted to cheating an exercise by holding their breath. This can have disastrous results for women and core exercise.

Continence is another job for which the core is responsible. The Pelvic Floor muscles are also not typically considered to be part of the core muscle system. Many women believe that losing their continence is just a fact of life. This is not a truth. I want to repeat this over and over: *Incontinence is not just a fact of life.* There are reasons for incontinence later in life. But not in your twenties, thirties, or forties. Just because you had a baby doesn't mean you are doomed to be incontinent.

The core is actually a group of seven different muscles that work together to perform a lot of different functions simultaneously. Many women are told they need to start a core exercise program because they are having core trouble. Some women develop core trouble when they start a core exercise program. Either way, it is extremely disappointing and frustrating to invest the time and energy into something that is supposed to be healthy and have it turn into more problems. Training the core is not like training any other set of muscles in the body. Starting at the wrong level with bad technique can lead to problems for some women.

Why Listen to Me?

I have been a physical therapist for thirty years, and my practice primarily deals with chronic pain. Chronic back pain, neck pain, pelvic pain, hip pain, head pain—you name it. That is what I like to treat. The reason I like that patient population is that every case is unique. To make a difference for a patient as a therapist, you must figure out what is missing.

Many different body issues stop working like they are supposed to for various reasons. The core muscles are extremely complex. Most people assume all you need to do to "fix" a back problem is to do the "Top Twenty Core Exercises." Though that may be true for certain cases, it is certainly not true for all.

Having seen thousands of patients with various types of chronic pain, I can estimate that 70 percent of them have a component of core dysfunction contributing to their problem. Notice that I said "dysfunction" and not "weakness." That's because there is more to the core than the Six-Pack muscle, and there are other types of problems besides weakness.

I would also estimate that the majority of this 70 percent are women. Women have to contend with a lot of challenges that are not a factor for men and that tremendously affect their core muscles. There are life events that cause big changes in one or more of the core muscles, and the "Top Twenty Core Exercises" program will not specifically restore what's missing. The end result can be worse than the existing problem.

The Only Constant in Life Is Change

Bodies change. Bodies change with age and bodies change with major life events. Nobody gets out for free (even though it seems like some people do). Many life events alter the way the body works. The most obvious one for women is having a baby. Your body is never the same after having a baby. It's not just about the changes in belly appearance. There are lots of ways your body has to adapt to accommodate growing a baby: The rib cage changes, the pelvis tips differently, the joints become more lax. These kinds of changes can set women up for having a lot of problems as they age.

Other life events include becoming an adult and getting a real job with real responsibilities. Having to spend most of your waking hours at a desk in front of a computer is a big change from spring break and summers off. This is huge for posture problems. That old saying "If you don't use it, you lose it" is so true here. Hips get stiff when they are flexed in a chair most of the day. Backs slump and shoulders roll forward. As a result, the core changes.

Stressors that manifest from work and homelife take a toll on posture as well. Emotional energy is very much reflected in how we feel compelled to comfort ourselves. The inevitable forms of loss and heartbreak, such as losing a loved one, weigh heavily on us. We drop our postures inward to protect a heavy heart. This certainly contributes to core changes.

Health conditions can have a big impact on how the core works, especially if they involve the lungs. Struggles with breath, like asthma or any other type of chronic obstructive disease, cause the Diaphragm to work differently. The Diaphragm has to flex and work harder, which puts a lot more pressure through to the Pelvic Floor. A major risk factor for organ prolapse in women is anything that causes a chronic, constant cough.

A variety of other health conditions cause changes in how the core muscles work. Any pain from any organ will cause the Inner Core muscles to relax and ease their tension in order to decompress that organ. Bloating and chronically excessive gas are painful and also need more space to be comfortable. This results in the core muscles letting go of tension to decompress. When the core lets go too often, it loses its muscle memory.

Accidents are the most traumatic and unpredictable life events. Any trauma involving the spine will cause big changes in the core. Imagine trying to recover from an accident that requires you to get your core strength back when you also have a two-year-old toddler and asthma. Imagine how awful it would be to develop incontinence because your core rehab program does not take all this into account.

Other changes in the body are simply related to getting older. This is true for all of us, but women have special considerations. A big part of our aging process is menopause and its accompanying loss of estrogen. This can cause huge changes for us. Bones get brittle, along with joints and connective tissue. It becomes harder to manage weight gain and keep up with muscle tone.

All these factors are important considerations for how to exercise, yet the "Top Twenty Core Exercises" program is designed for just one body. When I am directing a woman's rehabilitation program, I must take into account all the health issues the woman is dealing with. I also want to know her entire medical history. What accidents has she had? How many children has she carried? All this information is unique to every individual, and no body is the same as another body. This is the core truth I want to share in this book.

"Change" Is Another Word for "Opportunity"

The changes that come with age and life events can be hard to cope with, but there is something to be said for a good challenge. It's truly an opportunity to learn how your body works and to know just how to take care of your Lady Business for the rest of your life. If you never have a problem, then it's just not as meaningful.

You would think that in this day and age, there would be easy and accurate solutions that actually work for everything that ails. It's kind of like that annoying commercial advertising a drink that melts belly fat. We are still having to sift through nonsense to get to the heart of information. If it seems too good to be true, it likely is.

The good news is that there is hope for change. At any age, with any problem, there is hope. Your body is made of cells, and when you know how to load those cells, you will get a change. Strengthening your core is like growing a plant: If you give it the right light and water, it will grow new cells and change. You will become stronger.

When it comes to your core, please don't "Just Do It." You must do it well. It really is easier for men to change how their bodies work, even with age. Most of them can just step into an aggressive core training exercise program and move forward with no problem. Some do run into trouble with this approach, but they rarely realize it. This is mostly due to overtraining one set of muscles (the Six-Pack) and creating an imbalance of the core.

To get your core under control and be healthy for successful aging, you need to know what you are doing and how your body is working. If you don't, then your trainer should. Or your therapist. Or your coach. Everybody training bodies should understand how to assess the different parts of the core. It's not just seeing how many sit-ups you can do or how far you can reach. There is more to core fitness than that.

You need to meet your body where it is at. There is a rehab process to these things. First, you must establish what has happened to the body. For example: What ailments have caused what change in the relevant parts? How has the body compensated for these issues? Are you compensating because you are too tight in one or more core muscles? Is it truly a weakness problem or a combination of issues? What needs to change first? Without answering these questions (and others I'll pose throughout this book), jumping into a core training program unaware may just reinforce your compensation.

Don't Subject Your Complex System to Simplistic Fads

Exercise performed incorrectly can cause more harm than good. In the last twenty years, scientists have uncovered some truths about how each one of the core muscles works both individually and as a group. The core is complex, and it is very easy to end up with an exercise program that causes more problems than solutions—especially for women. Many women are pushed into a core training program that is simply too hard for a start, and then they are made to feel bad about themselves because they cannot "keep up."

I have seen many "core fitness" programs come and go. Some people do benefit from these programs, but many experience either no change or, even worse, more problems. There seems to be an aggressive attitude associated with core training. Women are told to push hard to feel the burn in their belly. One patient told me that a trainer actually screamed at her when she dropped out of a deep squat pose because she was leaking. When she explained to the trainer why she dropped, the trainer told her that leaking was okay and was a sign that she was finally working hard enough.

Another patient told me that she experienced a severe pain and spasm of her back muscles while working a plank maneuver during a fitness class. When she was able to stand and walk out, the trainer told her not to come back and that there was "something really wrong" with her that "needed professional help from somewhere else"!

At least that trainer gave the patient some advice that made sense. That patient did have something wrong that needed help. Whereas it wasn't as catastrophic as the trainer made it sound, that particular patient just needed some mobilization and stretching of her groin muscles so that she could achieve the proper position for a plank. Everything worked out okay for that woman, but this situation illustrates that the embarrassment of failing while trying to do something considered simple is a huge barrier. Many women feel that an initial inability to do something is their body's failure that can't be changed, so they choose to never get help.

There are important consequences of inappropriate core exercise management. There is a span of negative responses to core exercise that ranges from extreme to totally ineffective—to no change in muscle function. This range of responses is relative to the level of dysfunction within the core system itself, as well as to the health of the body. In other words, there is a variety of aspects of health to consider when prescribing core exercise.

Reasons You May Struggle

There are multiple reasons why women develop problems with their core muscle system. Changes in how a muscle works occur for many different reasons. These can include traumas, overuse injuries, having babies, and various disease processes. Some of these issues will also affect the muscle system of men, but there are significantly more issues that change the way a woman's body works.

Change in core muscle function has many consequences, one of which is a loss of support and control of the rib cage, spine, and pelvis. This kind of change in muscle function results in less stability of the bones in different postures, as well as an increase in shearing between the bones as we move. Over time, this instability of bone support will lead to inflammation developing, which causes pain and contributes to the vicious cycle of chronic pain and ongoing loss of function.

Other consequences of diminished muscle function involve the organ systems. The function of continence completely relies on muscular control and how those muscles influence their pressure system. How the organ system is supported is affected by change not only in the abdominal wall and the Pelvic Floor, but also in how well we breathe.

Sara, Rita, and Helen had great outcomes. They were able to make momentous changes in their bodies and regain the control they needed in their lives. A thorough assessment of each of the individual core muscles revealed which muscle was weak and dysfunctional, along with what muscles were compensating. This process of specifically rehabilitating the underlying health dysfunction allowed these women to progress back into a more traditional core exercise program.

The aim of this book is to provide all women with a better understanding and knowledge of what the core muscles are and how they function. Women have particular challenges in terms of their body's health and should not be prescribed exercises without all considerations specific to a woman's needs.

All women need a comprehensive understanding of how the core muscle system responds to all aspects of their personal health. You can then apply techniques that control and shape your health by controlling and shaping your core. So join me on this journey into the core truths of your womanly body.

PART ONE

UNDERSTAND JUST WHAT YOU ARE DOING

CHAPTER 1

The Science Beyond Fads and Internet Advice

Thirty years ago, "core exercise" was not a thing. I can say this because, thirty years ago, I graduated from physical therapy school and the term "core" was never used. I never heard it used in a sentence, unless it was referring to an apple, for the first ten years of my practice. The concept of exercise for your trunk region certainly isn't new. Back in the day, if you were running a rehabilitation program for your patient with back pain, you taught them back exercises or abdominal exercises.

You would think therapists everywhere would be so happy that exercise for such an important part of the body has become popular. I have seen many claims to fame by promoting the ultimate core training program. You can't throw a proverbial stick at the internet without hitting at least fifty experts extolling the virtues of their special core program.

The problem is, these core training programs have become so extreme, they are causing problems for some people—specifically, women. I have analyzed and compared these programs, and it is amazing how many different versions of crunches and planks there are. These programs are based on many misconceptions, and people are being driven into believing that core exercise is supposed to be this extreme.

Despite all my research, I still cannot say where the term "core" actually came from—although I did gain an interesting perspective on the history of exercise fads. I was surprised to discover that one of the earliest fads in exercise was Jane Fonda's Workout in the 1970s. The '80s featured Richard Simmons "Sweatin' to the Oldies," then the '90s saw Billy Blanks's Tae Bo and the Total Gym, most famously endorsed by Chuck Norris and Christie Brinkley. CrossFit (first launched by Greg Glassman) and Spinning (Mad Dogg Athletics' line of indoor bicycling products and classes) were big hits in the new millennium, which has now given way to Beachbody's P90X and Insanity.

What I observed about this progression of exercise fads correlates with how core training has evolved. Exercise has become extremely aggressive. There seems to be a huge misconception that exercise has to be very strenuous and ridiculously hard in order for it to be beneficial for the body. There is no physiological basis for this, and it is one of many beliefs promoted by people selling a product.

This trend in exercise aggression caught my attention as I started to hear from my patients how they would start an exercise program that caused them to get hurt. It is very hard to reeducate people (especially men) once they've adopted the belief that something is good for them. I became very interested in examining CrossFit when I read a study claiming that 80 percent of young women participating in it were incontinent. Then I saw an article that quoted a gynecologist saying this was okay. This is not okay. These are young women damaging their bottoms for the love of the sport, and they are being reinforced to do it. That is not okay.

Here is a core truth: No woman over the age of thirty-five who has given birth should just go to a Pilates or a CrossFit class or try any core training without first having their core muscle coordination checked out.

Why Core Training Isn't Simple

There are very few information sources that explain accurately how the core manages the body's internal pressure system. I want to offer a resource for women that accurately explains how these muscles work, specific to all of their different responsibilities, to help you avoid many problems.

One of the hardest things to explain in therapy is core muscle control and Pressure Mechanics. The core is different from any other group of muscles that work together to control a set of bones. Here's why: The entire organ system lives within this group of muscles.

Knee muscles only have to control a hinge movement of the bones. Hips and shoulders consist of a ball-and-socket pivot controlled by muscles. It's not that these muscle groups aren't interesting or challenging; they just aren't as complex as the core. The core muscles have additional responsibilities that are important to consider.

The organ system is full of fluids and air. It is pressurized, and the core muscles influence and manage that pressure. These muscles have to do double-time work compared to what is required of other muscle systems. The core is responsible for holding and moving the bones of the spine, pelvis, and rib cage, as well as supporting the organs, breathing, and managing continence. That's not just double time; that's quadruple times the amount of work!

For a system that is so important and that accomplishes so much, the most unfortunate aspect of the "free expert advice" on the core that is so easily accessible online is that it convinces people that an extreme level or intensity of exercise is the gold standard, that exercise has to feel that way and be that aggressive in order to do any good. The result is that when a patient with an overly clenched Pelvic Floor or External Oblique presents in my clinic, it is a hard sell to get them to let go of what they have already been sold on and do things differently.

Core exercise is not a one-size-fits-all enterprise. Not everyone should start at the same level. What's profoundly frustrating for actual experts is the lack of actual scientific foundation on which these core exercise recommendations are based. So I want to discuss the most popular fitness theme as it applies to your core muscles.

"You Have to Load It to Grow It"

It's true—you do have to load your muscles, bones, and connective tissues in order to maintain your body's health and fitness. All those electrical devices promising you can get rock-hard abs lying on your couch while getting zapped are selling lies. It doesn't work that way. You do need to get up and do some cardio, stretch your body, and move some resistance to keep your body working well. Anytime something isn't working well, consult with an expert in order to recover your working parts.

Anybody in the business of advising others on how to change their physical body should have a good working understanding of the growing zone. I like to call this the "Baby Bear Zone." This is the zone where the muscles and connective tissues are given just enough load, reps, and sets for a growth response. Not too much and not too little! Like Baby Bear, not too hard and not too soft.

The Baby Bear Zone is where the muscles and tissues respond to the exercise and get more control and flexibility, ultimately growing stronger. Fitness experts have known for decades that muscles and connective tissues will change depending on how much work they are required to perform. This goes both ways. If you don't use a muscle very much, then it atrophies and gets smaller and weaker. If you use a muscle, it will plump up, look fuller, and get stronger. If you overwork the muscles and connective tissues with too much load, you will get tendonitis, bursitis, or other muscle problems.

There are formulas for how this works. The main formula for developing strength is taking a percent of the maximum the muscle can do and structuring a certain amount of repetitions into a number of sets. One example is using an arm curl for getting stronger biceps. Let's say that the arm can curl a maximum of twenty pounds. A good strength program for growing that biceps is to work that arm curl with fifteen or sixteen pounds for ten to twelve repetitions for three sets. Science tells us that this formula will result in a stronger arm curl and bigger biceps in about three to four months.

What many people tend to do is guesstimate where they are and just pick a weight that makes sense to them. This is usually based on what the friend is doing next to them in the gym. Or what the trainer tells them to do—which may or may not be the same starting place for all of that trainer's clients. Then they pump that weight until they are completely exhausted with the idea that they have to tear that tissue down for the body to regrow it bigger and better. Unfortunately, the body doesn't quite work that way.

Using a formula is a reliable, safe way to work the arms and the legs, but it's not necessarily reasonable to use a formula with the core.

The core is a group of seven different muscles that rely on one another to do a bunch of different jobs simultaneously. Figuring out how much load to start with gets really tricky. Plus, you have a multitude of movement directions to choose from. The core works three-dimensionally and needs all groups to be balanced in all directions. This is why, for the core, you must consider how the entire body coordinates your exercise movements.

Coordination Is Key to the Core

There is a foundation of synchronization going on with every movement we make. The simple act of doing an arm curl to move weight is more than just bending the elbow. The muscles of the shoulder must stabilize the arm to hold steady for the movement of the elbow. The wrist has to grip the weight. Both the shoulder and the wrist must adjust their grip and tension levels depending on where the elbow is in its curling action. It is a different action of the shoulder and wrist to hold for the lift versus grip for the lowering of the weight.

What I'm describing is *coordination of muscles in a movement*. People get very focused on the action result of the movement—lifting the weight—but forget that the rest of the body is also coordinating for that action to happen. The challenge of coordination becomes more obvious when learning a new activity. It takes a bit of time for the body to learn the entire action and build it into its memory bank.

When learning a new exercise, it's a prime time for injuries to happen, especially if the exercise load is too high. If the movement is new or even something that isn't done on a daily basis, then the brain and muscles have to sort out how to do the movement and then practice it, so it is maximumly efficient.

So an arm curl really isn't a good example of how this kind of injury can occur, mostly because arm curling is something that everybody does all the time. You can't lift a fork without curling your arm. Doing a plank is a better example. It's not something that everybody naturally does every day and certainly not while lifting a fork.

Planking is more than an abdominal exercise. It's the coordination of arm muscles working to hold elbows straight and shoulders stabilized, while the abdominals are holding the rib cage in alignment with the pelvis, and the leg muscles are holding their joints straight and neutral. That's what's going on with the bones, but there is something else that is also supposed to be happening at the same time. Breath. Breath work is core work as well. That's a lot to coordinate at first, and it generally feels unnatural, as well as really hard, to breathe while holding a plank.

The first thing most people do while planking is hold their breath. In fact, they resort to breath holding with most challenging core exercises. This breath holding then becomes the habit for doing all of the exercises, and most trainers let it go. Holding breath not only becomes the habit with all core exercise, it becomes a huge problem—especially for women. This is a great example of skipping the coordination part and rushing to the strength portion. When women develop the habit of breath holding with every move, they create a lot of trouble for their internal pressure and organ system. This is just one example of how easy it is to underestimate the impact of core exercise.

A good therapist, trainer, or coach will understand that there are a lot of actions and coordination going on with any movement of the body. There has been a great deal of interesting research in the past twenty years that reflects this truth. When you lift your arm, what's the first muscle group that is activated? The Inner Core muscles. The Inner Core refers to the innermost muscles of the core. This group of muscles is activated first and is immediately followed by the Outer Core, which is then followed by the muscles of the arm. All of these muscles are active and adjusting throughout the full movement action. This is the same pattern for the leg movement. Specialists know that the core muscles are involved with all activity of the body. This is why they are so vital. But another thing we underestimate is the uniqueness of each and every body doing the workout.

Meet Your Body Where It's At

The challenge in starting a core program is matching the exercise demand to the weakest link in your body. This is hard to figure out. This is also the piece that has fallen by the wayside in the trending of exercise fads. The "Top Twenty Core Exercises" start people at the toughest level of exertion. This is not good body training. This is not good coaching. Maybe a body can compensate through thirty minutes of planking. Maybe that will work for two or three weeks of exercising. Is it worth it to find out that it wasn't the right place to start? Is it worth having to recover from a bout of tendonitis or a disc herniation or incontinence?

My main goal with this book is to inspire you to participate in the full range of core exercises, not just the extreme stuff. Don't get me wrong: It's fine to do CrossFit if that's a personal goal. I have a seventy-year-old patient right now who has rheumatoid arthritis. She does CrossFit twice a week. I encourage her to keep it up because she is doing it well, her body is well coordinated for it, and she has a good trainer. She is a great example of a woman who has carried a baby and has a significant medical issue but has worked at restoring her core coordination.

Maximum Contraction Equals Maximum Overload

The extremes cater to the belief that maximum contraction is the only thing that is good for the body. That ideology will get some people in trouble. I have another patient who is very devoted to her Pilates classes, and I am determined to motivate her in another direction. The Pilates studio she attends is particularly aggressive in how it encourages participants to exercise. At this studio, women are directed to hold their low back in a pelvic tilt to "imprint," clench their Pelvic Floor and all of the abs, then wave the rest of their body parts around.

This kind of exercise instruction teaches one level of coordination, which is max gripping and clenching. The core muscles are not meant to work 100 percent clenched all the time. People participate in this kind of grippy exercise and get the idea that they are supposed to hold their bodies in order to be healthy and safe. Unfortunately, it just creates other issues.

The patient I am trying to reeducate was referred to physical therapy because of significant pain in her higher back and pelvis. Her history of pelvic pain began after having her baby, and she thought Pilates would be good for it. It was . . . until it wasn't. She has completely recoordinated her Pelvic Floor into a constant high-tension gripping that is causing her to have even more pelvic and back pain. But that isn't the worst of it! Now she has a lot of pain with sex.

These are some of the toughest conditions to work through because it's all about reestablishing the right muscle memory and coordination. It takes time and patience with your body. I have found that healing is more effective when you understand why you need it. So let's get to the truth about what the core muscles are.

What Are the Core Muscles?

There are almost as many ways of describing what the core muscles actually are as there are plank positions. It is somewhat entertaining to hear and read "experts" instruct people in what they believe to be the key core muscles. They bring a tremendous amount of attention to the Six-Pack muscles as well as to the Gluteus muscles because they are stuck in the "Buns of Steel" and "Abs of Steel" era. They sell what motivates people in terms of improving their appearance, not what restores health to the body. So I'll describe your core muscles in a way that supports your health.

The core is the group of muscles that attaches to the bones of the rib cage, spine, and pelvis. This includes the Rectus Abdominis, External and Internal Obliques, Transversus Abdominis, Erector Spinae, Multifidus, Diaphragm, and Pelvic Floor. These are the primary muscles that hold the bones of the spine and pelvis together and upright against gravity, among other things. I do not include the Gluteus muscles because they are butt muscles, and I do not include the Trapezius and Latissimus because those are shoulder muscles.

I divide these muscles into two groups that I like to call the "Inner Core" and the "Outer Core." The Outer Core group is made up of the Erector Spinae / Multifidus group, the Internal Oblique, the External Oblique, and the Rectus Abdominis. The Outer Core muscles are the more powerful movement-based muscles. This group of muscles moves the bones and supports the actions that generate more power, such as lifting, pushing, and pulling.

The Inner Core group consists of the Diaphragm, the Transversus Abdominis, and the Pelvic Floor. It helps to understand that the muscle for breathing and the muscle for continence are also considered core muscles. The Inner Core muscles are the true multitaskers. They perform the basic functions of breathing and continence while also holding the bones of the spine, pelvis, and rib cage together.

These two groups of muscles rely on each other. If the Inner Core has any weakness, then the Outer Core has to compensate. Now let's dive deeper into what happens in a woman's core.

Lady Business

Everyone knows that a strong core is good for your back. What that actually means is that when all of these muscles are working well, your bones are working well. A core problem is more than just a muscle problem. It's a problem that impacts how your internal pressure system works. These problems are not just about muscle weakness. A problem with the core could be anything that is not working well with any or all of the bones. That means back pain, pelvic pain, neck pain, rib pain.

Then there is that other set of problems with the core, the problems that are more difficult to understand. The problems with pressure and pressure on the organs. As I shared earlier in this chapter, there is a whole set of organs that lives in the middle of the bones and muscles of the core. Those organs rely on Inner Core muscles to work well and do their job. If the Inner Core isn't working well, then you experience a problem with Lady Business.

Women are far more likely than men to have core muscle–related problems. I can trot out all the epidemiological studies that prove this, but that would become boring. Suffice it to say that women have more troubles with this area and that these kinds of troubles affect how well we age.

You see, a muscle problem with the core muscles is not the same as a muscle problem anywhere else in the body. It's not the same as a knee problem or a shoulder problem. Knee and shoulder problems require muscle work, just like the core; however, it is a lot easier to pick up a set of exercises for these body parts and do them without making your problem worse. Muscle problems with other joints in the body are more or less the same for men and women. The evaluation done for a man's knee problem is the same evaluation done for a woman's. The exercises for a man's shoulder problem are more or less the same exercises for a woman's shoulder problem.

A core muscle problem is different because those muscles control not only bones, but also the organ system business. This is extremely important to understand because, if you want to feel good through the years, you need to take care of all your body parts. That is the key to aging successfully. Successful aging entails keeping your body moving well through the later decades and feeling pretty good most of the time.

There is a fairly specific list of organ problems that can arise when the core muscles are not working well. These problems include incontinence, organ prolapse, constipation, and loss of lung capacity. Some men have some of these issues, but it is not the same as it is for women because women have a different-shaped pelvis, a different bottom, and estrogen. The Lady Business is different.

There Is Hope

These are exciting times because we know so much more than we did when I got out of school thirty years ago. We know so much more about how to target exercises so they are very specific to the task at hand. We understand the principles of *neuroplasticity*, which is how the brain and the nervous system work, so we can do a better job training coordination. We know why it is so important to consider what muscle is loaded to make the task better. It is far more effective to be specific to a problematic muscle than to randomly exercise for an uncertain outcome.

Now we know all about the internal pressure system and how it affects Lady Business. Back in the day, when incontinence problems occurred, there wasn't enough information to fix them. Sure, certain types of incontinence responded well to what we knew to do at the time; we just weren't as effective as we are now with all the different types of incontinence. Plus, we know more about what contributes to creating problems with incontinence.

Today there is a much greater understanding of the various health conditions affecting the core muscle system. For example, we now know that Inner Core changes in an asthmatic female can lead to organ prolapse—key information for core training. Another example is understanding that IBS changes the way the Inner Core muscles are activated.

We know more about how to avoid creating new problems when treating existing problems because we know to restore coordination before strength. The days of "muscling through" exercise must fade away. This is so important for women. Muscling through to be competitive or to keep up with men generally leads to no good.

Finally, we know more about successful aging. Women are not doomed to spending their final years bed-bound in diapers. Other changes in the body, like humpbacked postures and stiffness, cause balance problems that result in falls and fractured hips. These can be prevented. One of the key ingredients for successful aging is regular, consistent exercise. Exercise or physical activity has shown to be effective in prevention of heart disease, stroke, chronic respiratory disease, cancer, and diabetes—as well as in managing and reducing anxiety and depression. We need to maintain the strength of all our body parts so we can be strong enough to do all the things required to take care of life. This is true for both men and women from around the age of thirty-five onward. As we get older, we tend to accrue injuries and other health issues that affect the musculoskeletal system. "Physical activity" is a pretty broad term that includes all forms of exercise, and core exercise training is high on the list of what's most valuable for health.

Research is the best tool for revealing truths and what approaches really make a difference. While the trends reflect what we know about why exercise is good for us, who decided that exercise needed to become so aggressive and demanding? What scientific health organization released protocols that support this attitude? The research certainly doesn't reflect it. In fact, research that has examined what motivates people to exercise has produced some interesting results. One study revealed that men exercise for social and competitive reasons, whereas women are more focused on health reasons and weight management. One can therefore surmise that the trend toward aggressive, high-demand exercise may be driven more by appeal to the male attitude than by actual health benefits.

There is a lot of good news and excellent evidence that shows how Lady Business is supposed to work. It has contributed to better exercise and methods to go about restoring and improving your Lady Business. So let's focus on you.

It's Okay to Exercise Like a Girl

I ask you to develop realistic expectations about strength training for the best changes in your body. Start where your body is at, not where you want it to be. People have become too concerned that they're not doing enough to justify the time and work investment they're making, so they overexercise, which doesn't do them any good. I'm not saying there's no value in sit-ups or planks; I'm just noting that it's not an ideal place to start for many women. There is a range of load that leads to the best outcomes in terms of changing muscle strength. There is also understanding how all the different muscles of the core work.

In the past fifteen years, I have seen a significant increase in the number of patients who either develop back and neck pain or experience flares of pain in response to high-demand core exercises. The first challenge in helping these people is to readjust their expectations for exercise. There is quite a bit of trust building required at the beginning of a therapeutic relationship. You want to rely on therapists to base their recommendations on the most current evidence that research can offer.

This evidence is why a good therapist will evaluate all of the muscles of your core to make sure every muscle is doing its job. If you have been immersed in core guru propaganda, be ready for it to conflict with what a physical therapist recommends. Do not abandon therapy because the therapist's advice is incongruent with that of an internet "expert."

Both men and women are susceptible to changes in their core muscle function in response to pathological health processes. A good therapist will consider this for everyone when prescribing a core exercise program, particularly for women. We have touched on a few points that make women's cores different from men's, as well as the different challenges women face as we age. As these challenges accrue, they begin to compound upon one another and cause greater physical dysfunction and pain.

Imagine a forty-year-old woman who has had several babies and back pain ever since the last delivery. This woman also has asthma and a very mild case of occasional leaking, but only when she has waited too long to go to the bathroom. This woman should be managed completely differently than a forty-year-old man with asthma in terms of the core muscle exercise progression. She will require a complete assessment that evaluates each core muscle for its strength and flexibility. If she is mismanaged, then she will very likely experience significant increase in her back pain as well as less control over her continence.

Everyone wants to age successfully. Research shows that women tend to live longer than men, but women are somehow less likely to participate in any sort of structured exercise program continuously throughout their life. There seems to be an assumption that women should expect to naturally become frailer and bow into rounded postures until they can no longer stand straight. These aging ladies become incontinent and have very poor balance. Many end their lives bedbound because they lost their balance, fell, and broke their hip. There is a multitude of studies that show this is not the way things have to be.

We can change this physiological outcome at any point and at any age. The key is to invest the time and energy in getting the right start to an effective core exercise program. After you leave the internet experts behind, the next step is to learn the basic anatomy of your core.

CHAPTER 2

Anatomy of Core Muscles

There are a lot of expert opinions about which muscles of the body are considered core muscles. Some of these opinions are geared toward what is considered important by popular consensus, but that consensus is made by young people. Most people believe that the core muscles include the Rectus Abdominis, the Gluteus Maximus, and the Latissimus. Focusing on these translates into a ripped Six-Pack, a sculpted butt, and broad shoulders.

Every time I plan my core muscle rehabilitation program, I try to keep these kinds of beliefs and opinions in mind. I also am aware that many people have inaccurate assumptions about where their core muscles actually are. This is why I begin every patient program with an anatomy educational moment. I pull out my iPad and start up one of my favorite anatomy apps that stacks up the different muscles of the body by layers. This way, I have confidence that my patient has an accurate perspective on just where these muscles live in the body and what they do.

The value of a good anatomy educational moment became very evident to me early in my practice. I was surprised by my assumptions. One specific patient had some very strong ideas about her anatomy—this wasn't the surprise, because she was an art teacher at the local university. Artists have a certain amount of education in anatomy in order to create accurate images of the body. My surprise arose from this patient's beliefs about her anatomy.

As I started to guide her through her initial exercises, she became quite agitated with me. The anatomy that I was explaining to her did not correlate with what she believed to be the truth about her body. She agreed with me that she was quite weak in the area I was targeting, but she had a different impression about just where those muscles were located. By the end of our session, I started to understand that she thought the core muscles were entirely within the outermost layer of the body immediately under the skin. She believed the fleshy, plump part of her belly was where the muscles lay. This made it hard for her to believe that the firmness of the muscles was deeper than that.

Over the years, many people have come to me thinking their muscles were nonexistent based on the way their belly feels. This belief leads to a sense of hopelessness that nothing can be done to change the body. There are a lot of mistaken ideas about core muscles and how they relate to the shape of the belly. Often, the shape of the belly has very little to do with the amount of *adipose tissue*, or body fat, there but, rather, with how the core muscles are working.

Core truths and anatomy are important for you to understand in order to regain control of your life and body. So let's get to the heart of this kind of knowledge through an anatomy educational moment. You must know where each muscle is and what it does in order to change it.

This anatomy educational moment might get a little overwhelming with all the Latin, and I know it's hard to keep track of what's what. But I've tried to distill the information down to the key essentials along with better ways to think about these muscles. So please bear with the official terms because they will lead to the nicknames that make more sense.

Keys to Understanding Your Anatomy

Here are a few key things to keep in mind that explain what you'll be seeing in the illustrations, coupled with some fun facts about anatomy, especially core muscle anatomy.

The red meat of the muscle never attaches directly to the bone. The red meat has to turn into a white, gristly tendon in order to attach to bone. Muscles appear to be red because they contain a lot of *myoglobin*. Myoglobin is what stores oxygen. All muscles require a significant amount of oxygen, but some need more than others, particularly muscles that have to work constantly through the day, like postural muscles. Tendons are white because their job is to hold the muscles' connection to the bone.

Muscles have a fiber direction that tells you what kind of action the muscle performs. Muscles consist of contractile elements that shorten and lengthen with tension. These contractile elements slide, then interlock. They interlock to hold a bone steady, which is called *isometric contraction*. They can also slide and lock, which is known as *isotonic contraction*. This sliding and locking tension takes place in the red, meaty part of the muscle.

All muscles are connected to a nerve that is their electrical source. Every muscle in the body is hooked into an electrical grid that lives in the brain. If the muscle isn't hooked into the nervous system, then the muscle can't be contracted. No nerve connection = no muscle contraction.

The core muscles are unique in that the contractile elements are arranged in broad sheets of muscles that end in expansion of white, gristly connective tissue called *aponeurosis*. This is different than the muscles of the arms and legs, which tend to be organized in more rope-like configurations. These broad sheets are required to control the spine, the cage, and the pelvis. That is a lot of territory to manage.

Core muscles have multiple demands that must be performed simultaneously. They can work this way because they are organized in layers. It is easier to talk about them and what they do by dividing them into two groups: the Inner Core and Outer Core. As first introduced in chapter 1, the Inner Core consists of the three internal muscles, and the Outer Core includes four muscles that layer over the Inner Core. Here, we'll go over these groups in more detail.

Intro to the Outer Core Muscles

The Outer Core muscles are more familiar to most people because they appear on almost all anatomy illustrations. The Outer Core consists of the External Oblique, the Internal Oblique, the Rectus Abdominis, and the Erector Spinae / Multifidus group.

The External Oblique originates from the front and lateral sides of the lower six ribs. This broad muscle runs downward and in toward the center to blend in with its aponeurosis to the *linea alba*. The lower muscle fibers end up attaching the pelvis. Note the fiber direction.

The Internal Oblique originates from the *iliac crest* of the pelvis underneath the External Oblique and rises up obliquely (hence the name) to blend in medially with its aponeurosis. The upper muscle fibers also attach to the lower four ribs.

I group the Internal and External Obliques together because they are designed to work as a unit. I call them "the Obliques" because their muscle fibers run vertically at oblique angles. The Obliques cover the front and side of the core. The red muscle fibers attach to the white aponeurosis. The Obliques' aponeurosis forms a pocket that supports the next muscle, the Rectus Abdominis.

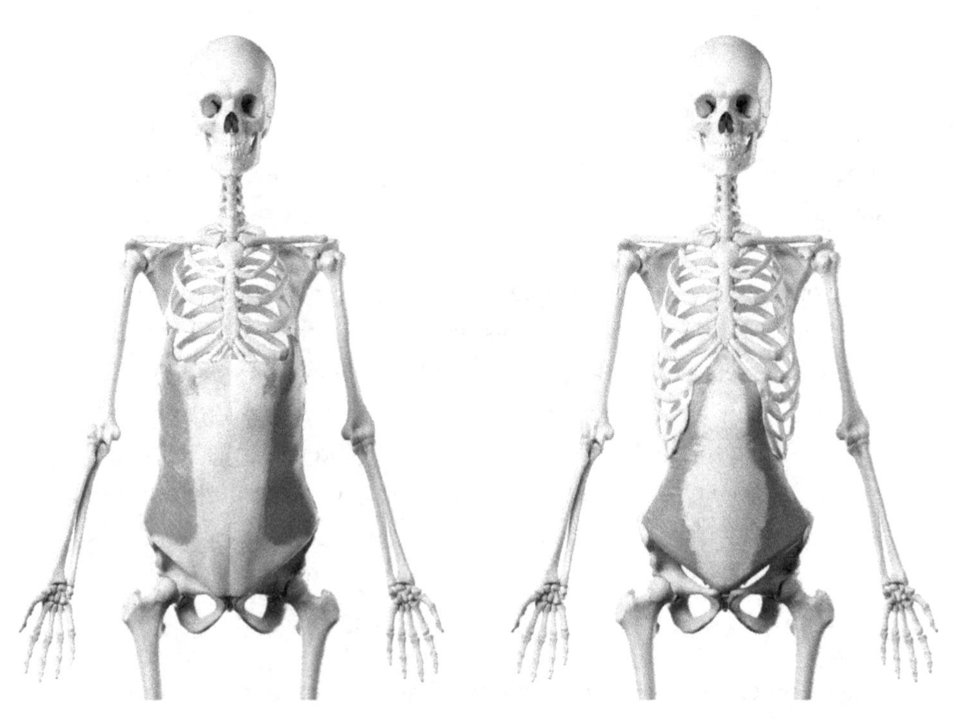

External Oblique (*left*) and Internal Oblique (*right*)

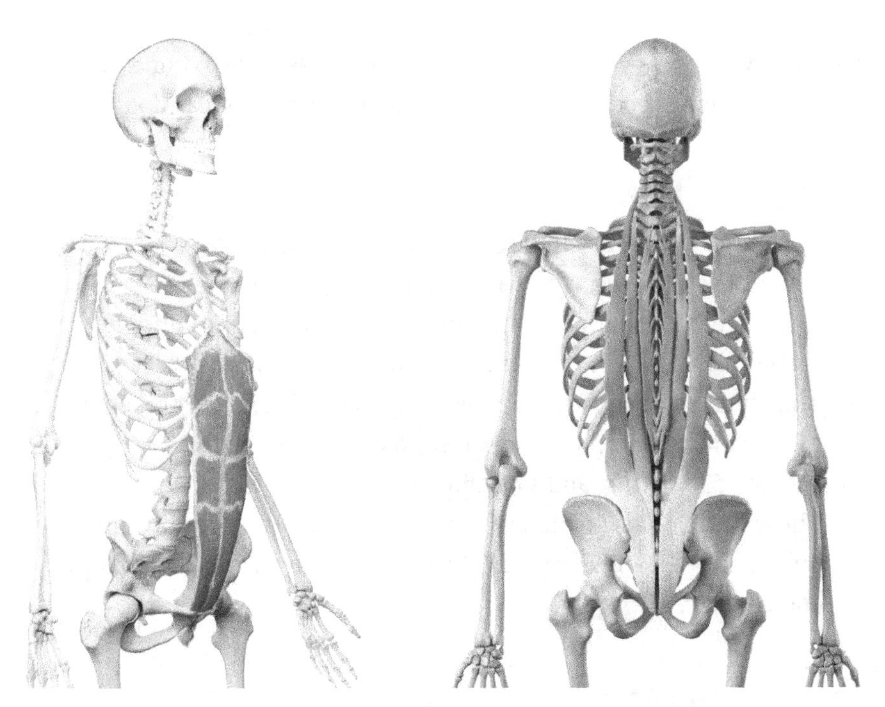

Rectus Abdominis (*left*) and Erector Spinae (*right*)

The Rectus Abdominis is a pair of long, flat muscular straps that extend from the lower sternum and inner part of the fifth, sixth, and seventh ribs down to the pubic bone. Both of these muscle straps are encased within the aponeurosis, and their unique action is to flex the spine.

I like to call this muscle "the Six-Pack"—mostly because that's what everyone else calls it.

The Erector Spinae / Multifidus muscles are grouped together because they control the back side of the spine with bending and tipping. The Multifidus are the deepest muscles and they attach from bone to bone. The Erector Spinae is a group of long, strappy muscles that overlap the Multifidus. These muscles run from the back side of the pelvis and connect throughout the bones of the spine up to the top of the thoracic and rib cage.

I call this group of muscles "the Back Strap." I started referring to these muscles by this term because I have been working in Alaska for the last twenty-five years, and many folks in Alaska like to hunt—everybody here knows where the back strap is on a moose or caribou.

Outer Core Facts

- The Outer Core muscles are vertical connections between the upper spine and rib cage down to the lower spine and pelvis.
- The Outer Core supports and holds the stack of bones upright with vertical tension, kind of like a guy wire system on a baby tree.
- The Outer Core muscles are also very dynamic and control a lot of movement actions of the bones, such as bending forward and backward, twisting, and side tipping.
- These muscles also generate large torques of power for pushing, pulling, lifting, and carrying. They are the movers, reachers, lifters, and carriers.

Intro to the Inner Core Muscles

The Inner Core muscles provide a base of connection for the Outer Core muscles to work over. This group includes the Diaphragm, the Transversus Abdominis, and the Pelvic Floor. This group of muscles is the ultimate multitasker. As a unit, these muscles work together to form a pressurized core of muscle support for the internal organs, to connect and stabilize the bones, to breathe, and to provide continence.

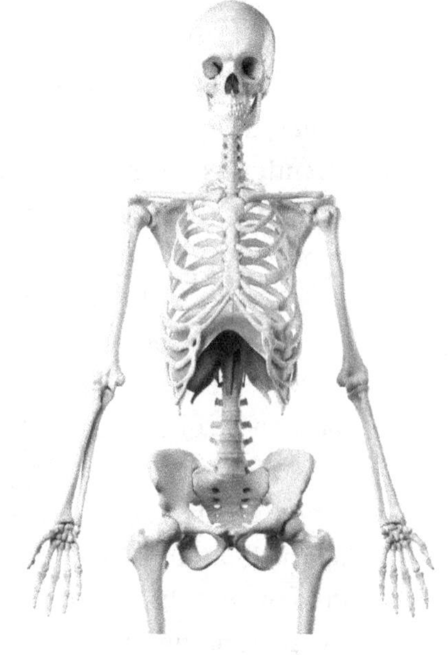

Diaphragm

The Diaphragm is the top muscle of the Inner Core. It attaches all the way around the periphery of the base of the rib cage. Its muscle fibers rise up from the cage base to meet in a central white tendon forming a dome-shaped muscle that lives within the cage. The lungs and heart rest on the top of this muscle. When the Diaphragm contracts in order to inhale air, the muscle fibers pull the central tendon downward while expanding the rib cage at the same time. It is this downward pull with expansion that draws air into the lungs.

I like to call the Diaphragm "the Breather muscle" because it is the main muscle that drives breath. This muscle also has other functions that include postural connection and tension to stabilize the rib cage, as well as the bearing-down action needed for a bowel movement.

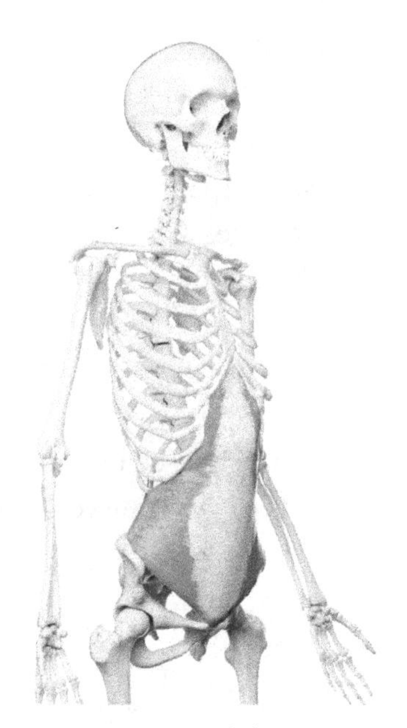

Transversus Abdominis

The Transversus Abdominis muscle lies under the Oblique muscles, which makes it the innermost muscle of the abdominal wall. It originates from three main areas: the iliac crest of the pelvis, the deep *fascia* or connective tissues of the back muscles, and the inside of the lower six ribs. The muscle fibers travel transversely around the side and front of the core to blend into its aponeurosis much like the outer Obliques do. Its main job is to function much like a corset for the body. It's more of a holder of the bones and organs than a mover. It also assists breathing by contracting and cinching in the abdomen to push the Diaphragm up to exhale air.

Some people like to think of this muscle as the corset, but I prefer to call it "the Encasement muscle." Its muscle action encases the organ system, helps the Breather muscle with breath control, and connects the stabilizing support for the cage, the spine, and the pelvis. It's actually the muscle we use to talk and to sing. We inhale air with the Breather but then use the Encasement muscle to push the air through the vocal cords.

The Pelvic Floor is an interesting configuration of small muscles layered together that form a hammock shape. The sphincters for the urethra and the anus, as well as the vagina, are embedded within this group of muscles and rely on its strength in order to work well. This muscle hammock connects the tailbone up to the pubic bone and lives on the inside of the sitz bones.

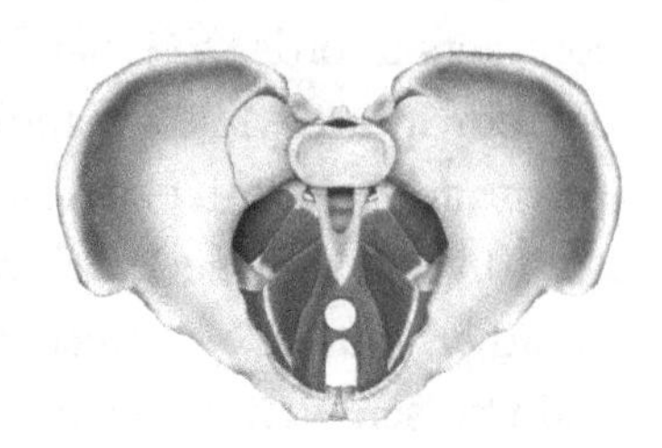

Pelvic Floor

It's easiest to call this group of muscles simply "the Floor." This muscle group supports the base of the pelvic bones as well as the bottom of the organ system, which includes the bladder, uterus, and rectum/colon. In addition to bone and organ support, the Floor controls both urinary and fecal continence in men and women. Obviously in women, it has the additional challenge of supporting the vagina and uterus. These muscles also contribute to assisting the Encasement muscle in exhaling by increasing tension and lifting to help the Transversus Abdominis push up the Diaphragm.

Inner Core Facts

- The Breather, the Encasement, and the Floor muscles are the horizontal core muscles. They connect the front to back and side to side of the core.
- The Inner Core muscles encase the organs and support them.
- The Inner Core muscles hold and maintain continence.
- The Inner Core movement actions are breathing, talking, singing, coughing, and anything that involves moving air.

Core Tensions

An accurate evaluation of the core muscles requires an understanding of what each of these major muscle groups is responsible for and how they work together. Cranking out a bunch of crunches and planks doesn't give you a rating of strength for the core; it only tells you how strong you are in one part of the core. This doesn't indicate how well the individual core muscles are functioning, and it doesn't provide a complete picture of how well the muscles are performing together.

The manner in which core muscles depend on one another was not completely understood until the past fifteen years. These muscles have a multitude of demands that they control for in a very symbiotic manner. They work together to hold the body upright. The Inner Core supports horizontally for the Outer Core to use its vertical advantage to bend and move the body. These muscles can accomplish all of these things because there is a tension relationship between each one of these muscles.

Imagine each muscle group as having its very own tension dial. Zero on the dial of tension is how much tension the muscle is holding when the body is lying down. It is the most relaxed state of the muscles. Level 1 is the baseline tension of the muscles. This is the amount of tension required to basically hold the bones upright and stacked when standing, sitting, and walking. The other end of the spectrum is Level 10. This is the maximum amount of tension that a muscle can reach. Tension levels ramp up and down this spectrum in order to accomplish actions like twisting, bending, and lifting.

When the body is not well trained and balanced in exercise, then it plays favorites with certain muscles. One of the muscle groups starts to dominate posture with its tension levels. When a tension imbalance sets in, then the posture is skewed and the bones' connective tissue starts to get strained.

One of my favorite patient memories in terms of problems with imbalanced muscle tension involves Alexa. Alexa was a bodybuilder and very successful in the competitive arena. She was twenty-five years old when I first met her and new to the sport of bodybuilding. Unfortunately, she did not have a very good coach. In fact, her "coach" was a friend of a friend who was actually a chiropractor and who thought he could properly guide this woman through the complex training process of developing that level of muscle.

There is a tendency for men to focus on training the muscles that they think are the most important and attractive. That translates into a seriously ripped Six-Pack, which is what Alexa developed. Alexa also had a significant amount of upper-back pain to go with those ripped abs.

When you break the muscles down into force vectors on the body, it is easier to visualize the tension relationship among all of the muscles. When the Six-Pack is overtrained in comparison to the other muscles of the core, its tension level is ramped up and higher than the others, making it hard to balance out. Higher tensions of the Six-Pack cause the rib cage to be pulled forward more, which puts a strain on the muscles of the Back Strap. This difference in tension levels strains posture and causes back pain.

This is a really good example showing how the tension levels of the Outer Core muscles affect one another. These tension imbalances also affect the Inner Core's job, but in a different way. The Inner Core works with the Outer Core to hold the bones. The Inner Core also has its own job of supporting organ function. It holds the organs, it maintains continence, and it breathes. The tension relationship among the Inner Core muscles is more strongly linked because they are in charge of the internal pressure system of the body.

Picture the organ system. At the top is the stomach and liver. In the middle is the small bowel and colon, and at the bottom is the bladder, uterus, and rectum. All of these organs are full of fluid and air. It's kind of like the organ system is one big water balloon. This water balloon is supported by the core muscles, with the Inner Core muscles handling the responsibility for how the whole system works.

This water balloon acts like any other fluid-filled vessel when something starts adding pressure down on it. High tension of the Six-Pack muscle causes more pressure to load down on the water balloon, which translates to more pressure on what lives at the bottom of the balloon—in this case, the bladder. The Floor of the Inner Core can support only so much pressure from the water balloon. Once that tension wears out the Floor, it can't hold continence and we leak.

This is a classic example of what can happen with muscle imbalances of the core. Muscle imbalances of high-tension Six-Packs as well as of Obliques override the capabilities of the Inner Core muscles. That translates into more pressure inside the water balloon.

Alexa was sent to me not only for her back pain; she was also experiencing a lot of pelvic pain and the beginning of incontinence trouble. She was losing control of her bladder on occasion, which was obviously becoming worrisome for her.

It was good that Alexa reached out beyond her coach to get help because she really needed it. It was important to educate her about how all of these muscles work together in order to teach her how to properly train the muscles. It is possible to have a ripped set of Six-Pack muscles but still be healthy with good continence and no back pain. It took about six months to redirect Alexa's program and restore her health.

So again: You can't evaluate the muscle strength and tension levels of the Inner Core with a crunch or a plank. All trainers and physical therapists should know and understand how to properly evaluate coordination and control of all the core muscles to safely coach core training for women. Lady Business is different than men's business. Men have a different Floor configuration to their urethras. From a clinical perspective, this means that adding more pressure to a man's Floor does not result in incontinence as easily as it can for women. Men also have a different shape to their pelvis.

Assessment of the Inner Core takes some training in terms of targeting the different functions of the Breather, the Encasement, and the Floor muscles. Additionally, it's important to understand the tension interactions that each of these muscles has on the organ system. I call this "the Pressure Mechanics." This term describes how the Inner Core muscles are doing their job for the body, how well they are supporting the internal pressure of the organs.

It takes time to implement a good core training program, and hopefully, your coach/trainer/therapist will guide you in the right direction. In order to change how the body is working, it is essential to first identify exactly what muscle and what action we hope to change, as well as the effect of this intended change on all the other muscles. I personally have found that women like to understand the why of things. There is an investment of time and energy in this process, and you get better results when you know why you are doing things.

Assessing the core muscles is all about understanding how each muscle interacts with the others. Each muscle of both the Outer Core and the Inner Core needs to be evaluated. All of these muscles impact the internal Pressure Mechanics, the internal pressure system of the body. This is critical to understand because the operation of the pressure system affects the health of our body and how well we age. A poorly managed system of pressure can result in severe dysfunction, pain, and misery. So now we'll look at how the Pressure Mechanics works.

CHAPTER 3

Essentials of Pressure Mechanics

The internal pressure system is one of the toughest systems to explain in women's health. It is so easy to get lost in the anatomy, and by the time you get to how it all relates to internal pressure, it's just a little too much to digest. Still, understanding how the internal pressure system is managed and controlled by the Inner Core system is key to a good recovery of core muscle control—not to mention prevention of developing a lot of really uncomfortable problems with Lady Business.

The three major muscles in charge of this area are very susceptible to changing how they hold tension in response to pain and other types of problems. Any one of these muscles can change the way they function, but the difference is so subtle that people rarely recognize the change.

I have found it easiest to explain and conceptualize the relationship between all of the muscles and the organ system by relating the dynamics in terms of everyday things. When you put all of these components in play, it makes understanding how the interactions work much easier. It also helps with understanding how to change a component that isn't working well. Here is a summary overview of the Inner Core muscles for easy reference.

Inner Core Muscles . . . Again

The Breather muscle: the dome muscle at the top of the core that contracts to flatten and spread in order to draw air into the lungs; furthermore, it supports, controls the base of the rib cage from the front of the spine, and bears down for bowel movements.

The Encasement muscle: the muscle that literally wraps around the body like a corset, connecting the base of the rib cage to the spine and the top of the pelvic bones.

The Floor muscles: the group of muscles shaped like a hammock that supports the base of the pelvis and maintains continence.

All three of these muscles act together to:

- Support and hold the bones of the rib cage, spine, and pelvis
- Support the organs of the body
- Breathe
- Maintain continence

Four Steps to Understanding Pressure Mechanics of the Body

1. We begin centrally within the abdomen by imagining the stack of organs and how they are grouped together. At the top of the stack is the stomach and liver. The middle part, which can be considered the largest part, consists of the small bowel and large colon. At the bottom, going from front to back, is the bladder, the uterus, and then the rectum. All of the organs are clustered around the main stem of blood vessels that is nestled against the front of the actual bones of the spine. All of these organs are filled with fluids, blood, and air. When you encapsulate this entire group, you'll recall, it functions a lot like a water balloon.

2. The Breather muscle covers the top of the water balloon and functions like an elastic plate.

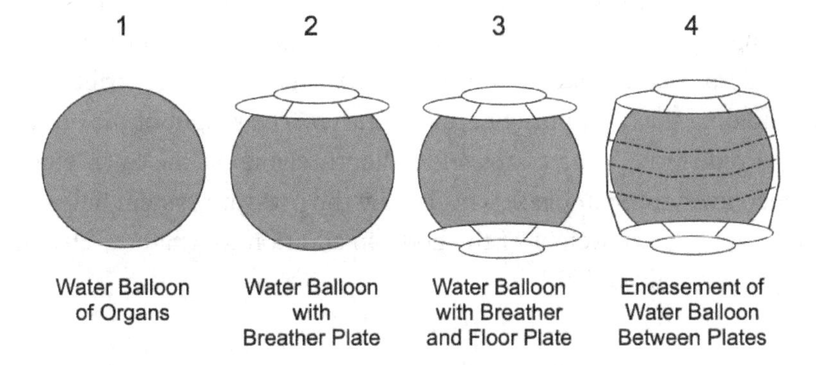

3. The Floor muscles also function like an elastic plate and sandwich the bottom of the water balloon with the top of the Breather plate.
4. The Encasement muscle wraps around the water balloon to encase it between the two plates.

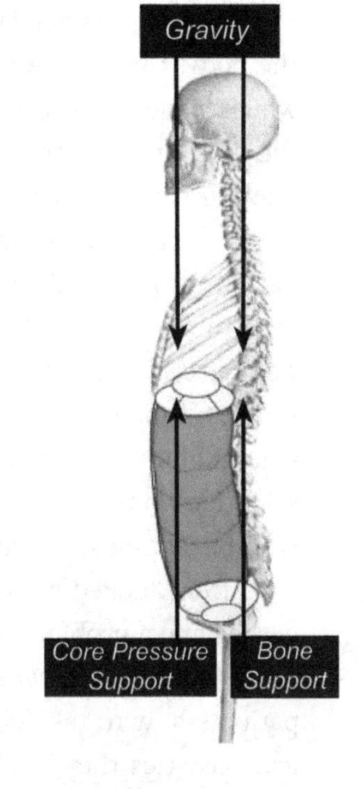

When you put tension through the Breather plate, it flattens and expands, creating a downward pressure on the balloon. When you draw in the Encasement, it squeezes and pressurizes the midsection of the balloon. When the Floor muscle plate contracts, it shortens, which flattens and creates an upward pressure on the balloon. And when all three muscles increase their tension levels and put a squeeze on the water balloon from all sides, the pressure inside the balloon increases.

All of these actions of muscle tension putting pressure on the water balloon happen within the body every day. These pressure changes are normal and subtle, but they're important. Every time we breathe, all three muscles are managing the pressure changes. Every time we lift something, all three muscles support the organs and bones for the additional weight. Every time we eat and digest, all three muscles take part in supporting the digestive process. Talking, shouting, singing, all involve the coordinative actions of these muscles.

This pressure system with its muscle support also contributes to just holding the body upright against gravity. The weight of the body is supported through the plates and balloon relying on the Encasement to keep everything in place. This is how the pressure system helps the bones hold all the weight of the body, in addition to whatever else the body might want to hold.

Pressure System Mechanics in Action

Obviously, the human digestive system is not organized in a ball and the Breather and Floor muscles are not shaped like plates, but the actions and relationships are there. It is a tough system to envision within your own body, but this metaphor provides the right kind of insight women need to understand how it works.

All therapists need to explain the body's mechanics in order to train the body. I wasn't very good at explaining these things ten years ago, which made it really difficult for me to help this young patient I had at the time—too young to be having the types of problems she was having. She was referred to me for pelvic pain, which was getting worse.

Her area of pain was centered over the right back side of the bony part of the pelvis. She was experiencing a lot of pain after walking more than thirty minutes. During the history part of the initial health questionnaire, she affirmed that she was having some problems with incontinence. When I asked her about this, she seemed surprised that it was a point of interest to me. In fact, she said, "Isn't that just a part of being an active woman?" I was a little stunned and asked her to explain where she got that idea, but she couldn't really say.

After I looked her over and did a few tests, it was obvious that she was having a problem with her right *sacroiliac joint*, the joint that links the pelvis to the lower spine. A big part of physical therapy is teaching patients how to take care of their injured areas to optimize the physical activities they really want to do. One of her favorite things that she really wanted to do was CrossFit, but it had become too painful to participate in.

We worked for several weeks with manual therapy and exercises to get her better stabilized. After she made good progress, it was time to look at the specifics of some of the exercises she wanted to be able to do in her CrossFit class when she went back. This is where I gained a much better understanding of not only her sacroiliac pain, but also her issue with incontinence. During one of our discussions, she explained to me that one of the trainers at her gym had helped her get better at jumping by taking in a big, deep breath and holding it while she jumped and landed. Then I understood. Breath holding is a common cheating strategy when we are not truly strong enough to rely on just muscle power. To understand how this pertains to this patient, we need to talk Pressure Mechanics and breath.

Inner Core Breath Mechanics

The pressure system is a very dynamic system in which tensions shift in response to how the body as a whole is loaded, as well as in response to breathing action. Using this model, we can show how the pressure system works with the simple action of breath:

Pressure Mechanics of Breathing

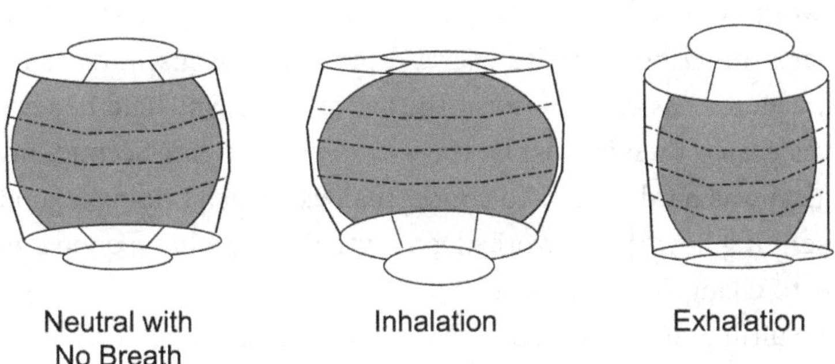

Neutral with No Breath | Inhalation | Exhalation

Inhalation involves the spreading and flattening of the Breather plate on the water balloon. As the breath increases, there is a downward pressure on the water balloon, which actually moves it as much as two centimeters. This movement of the balloon is guided and supported with an expansion of the Encasement into the Floor plate, which has to deepen to accommodate it. Many therapists describe the Floor muscle as a trampoline, and this is one of the reasons why.

This process reverses with exhaling breath. The Breather plate rises and deepens as the water balloon is lifted back up by the Floor plate with the help of the Encasement. It doesn't take a lot of work or tension for natural resting breath to happen. However, that changes with different physical demands. All of these muscles increase their action when we are working harder.

Imagine taking a big, deep breath and holding it in full while jumping and landing repeatedly. Think of how much force is driven into the Floor plate over and over by the water balloon. Remember, what is the bottom of that balloon? The Lady Business! This is a great representation of how the tension of what the body is doing, coupled with the high load on the water balloon, will cause excessive forces in an area that is not engineered to work like that. When this is going on over and over, our Lady Business suffers along with our continence. We will come back to this example over and over throughout the book because this dynamic is a big deal.

Back to my patient: I tried to convince her that all of that breath holding was creating a lot of high loading on her Pelvic Floor muscles, which in turn was affecting how both her pelvis and her continence were working. It was very difficult to convince her to change how she was performing her favorite exercise for two reasons. First, she just found it much easier to perform the action when she held her breath. If it was easier, then it must be the way to go . . . right? Second, my explanation was hard for her to conceptualize. I wasn't doing a good job of describing how things worked, so I wasn't giving her a good enough reason to change her approach.

She ultimately consulted with another therapist, and I never heard how things went for her. The frustration of my inadequacy stayed with me. I wanted to be a good therapist, but if you can't clearly explain how things work, you can't help remedy dysfunctional movements.

Pressure Mechanics and Posture

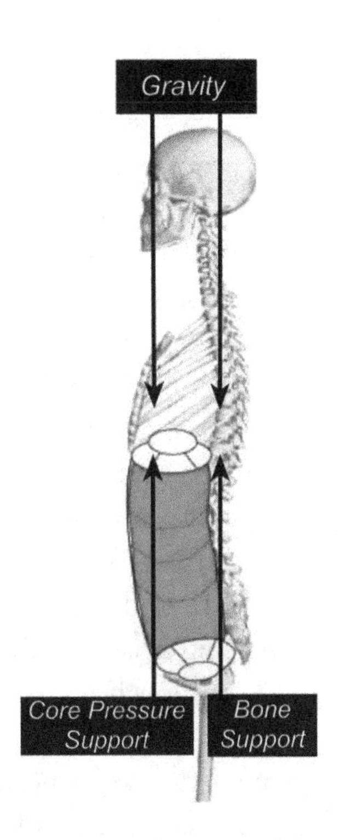

As I mentioned earlier, the body's pressure system is one of the mechanisms that holds it upright against gravity. In other words, there is a certain amount of load that goes through the core's plates, supported by the water balloon with the help of the Encasement. How the plates are able to distribute the load onto the water balloon is important in terms of the health of both the organs and the bones. Obviously, it is ideal to have a good distribution of load throughout the entire balloon.

It is important to remember that there are organs within the balloon that are used to a certain amount of body loading. In fact, some of the organs greatly benefit from loading and from the natural movement of the balloon with breath, which will be covered in more detail later. An optimal alignment of the plates along with the dynamic support of the Encasement will distribute the forces throughout the water balloon of organs, keeping everybody happy and moving.

Poor posture of the plates can have an unfortunate impact on organ function. The organs are just like any other tissue in the body in that too much pressure or loading can be detrimental, leading to pain and dysfunction. Poor posture of the plates also has an unfortunate impact on the entire musculoskeletal system. When the Inner Core cannot work well, other muscles must compensate, which results in tissue overload, inflammation, and pain.

This is important to keep in mind when considering all of the ways the Inner Core muscles can support the organs and the bones. Posture is a struggle, but it's a worthwhile endeavor, especially when you think of how our bodies age. Nothing gets easier as we get older. Optimizing the way the body works is a truly useful investment toward successful aging.

Posture Is Plate Alignment

Posture is without a doubt one of the hardest things to change. It's like all good habits in life—it's much easier to take the easy way out and just let it go. Once it's gone, though, it is aggravating to get back on track. We've all been told to "Hold your shoulders back" by Mom or someone else important in our lives. However, this is not a useful strategy. Shoulders do not hold the body upright against gravity. The core and the bones of the rib cage, spine, and pelvis do that.

Another tactic for optimizing posture is to get focused on maintaining a certain alignment of the head and spine bones. I frequently hear patients worry about pulling their head in and holding their back flat. Lots of women generate very high muscle energy in their efforts to keep their bellies pulled in. All of these efforts result in adding a lot of bracing tension to the body.

Although it's true that there is an ideal alignment of the bones, proper posture really has more to do with where the thoracic rib cage is in relation to the pelvis. One of the main jobs that bones have is to support weight. Rather than fretting over each individual bone, it is best to start with lining up the two parts of the body that are the densest with bone: the pelvis and the thoracic rib cage thorax cage.

This is the best place to start for two reasons. The Breather plate lives in the thoracic rib cage and the Floor plate lives in the pelvis. When these two plates are out of alignment, the pressure within the water balloon changes.

There is a whole host of consequences to changes in the pressure system, most of which manifest in that which lives within the water balloon of organs. These consequences are covered in greater detail in part two of this book. Understanding these consequences requires some knowledge of Pressure Mechanics.

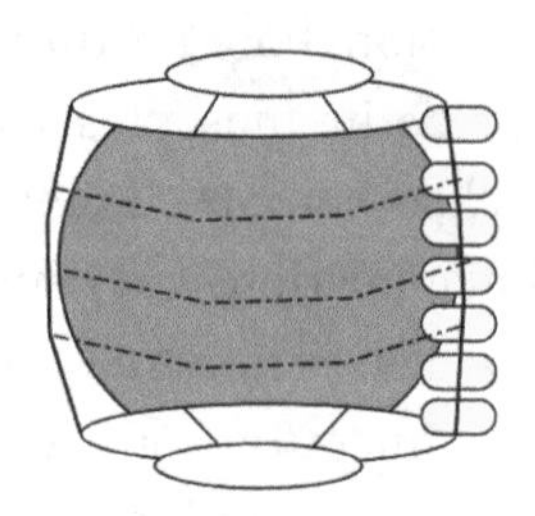

Sideview of the Pressure System

Posture gets sloppy in a variety of ways. Researchers have identified some of the most common changes in posture.

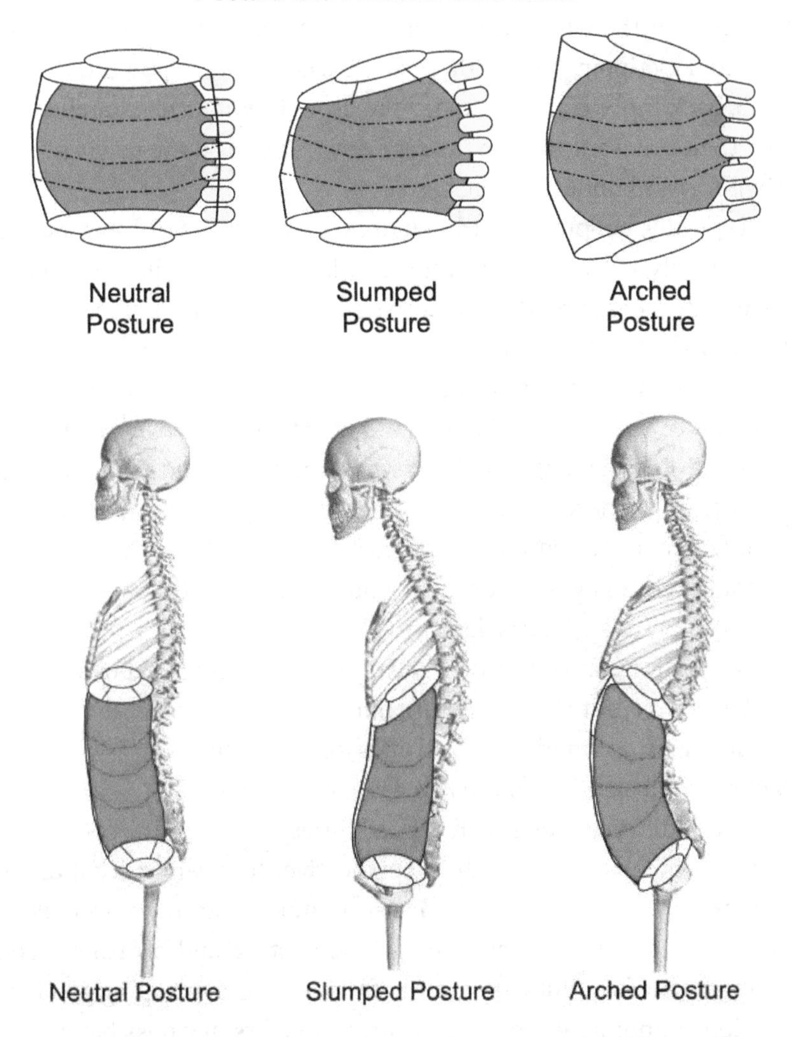

Slumped posture causes the top Breather plate to become tipped down and shifted backward relative to the Floor plate, which usually becomes somewhat tipped up. The arched posture orients the Breather plate forward and tipped up in relationship to the Floor plate, which is usually significantly tipped down.

These changes in plate orientation also impact how effective the Encasement muscle is in doing its job. This becomes a little more obvious when we move this pressure system model into an actual skeleton.

Optimizing posture always should begin with lining up the thoracic rib cage over the pelvis. If you have a slumped posture habit, it can be corrected by tipping up the thoracic rib cage thorax cage a bit, then the pelvis back more centrally under the cage. If you have an arched posture, then you want to drop the cage down and relax the pelvis so it can orient forward under its cage.

Typically, people are told to muscle up the pelvis or the shoulders, but the only thing that accomplishes is to exhaust the muscles and make body parts sore. If the focus starts with the cage and pelvis, then the head stacks up and the shoulders orient where they need to.

All of this is easier said than done, often because there is usually a weakness or stiffness that has evolved with bad habits over time. Sometimes the Encasement muscle has become weak, and sometimes the Back Strap has become too stiff. There is a myriad of medical conditions (many of which are discussed later in the book) that can also contribute to changes in how these muscles are functioning.

The body as a whole is designed to stand the test of time. It has a lot of capacity for compensation. As we get older, things happen, and we need to compensate in how we use our bodies. Unfortunately, compensations have a cost and nothing comes for free in life. This is what leads to muscle imbalances, and that is why I have a job.

The different roles and responsibilities of the entire core system make it difficult to keep it all in perspective. It is very helpful to have a structured program process so that no muscle starts to override the function of another muscle. Things like posture and breath are commonly overlooked, but they are the platform for developing good core function. Running, jumping, and lifting weights are possible and can continue to progress if the Inner Core's ability to control and support pressure system posture while breathing well meets the capacity for the Outer Core's strength and power demands.

CHAPTER 4

Truths About Core Strength and Core Control

There are a lot of assumptions about what core strength is and what having core strength will do for the health of your body. I get these kinds of questions every day from my patients. Sometimes it's difficult to answer them because some of the explanations can be confusing, especially if my patient has spent any time on the internet.

Is it important for the core to be strong? Yes.

Will my pain go away if I get my core strong? Maybe . . .

How strong should my core be? Hard to say. Depends on what you want to do.

Those are the short answers to some of the common questions. The longer, more accurate answers have actually cost me business because the term "core strength" is so misunderstood. When I talk to patients about their core muscle function, I no longer use the term "core strength." I talk about "core muscle control." There is a lot of misleading information about what the core muscles need for health, and getting to the truth of the matter requires defining the difference between strength and coordination, as well as clarifying how they interact.

Here are more specific answers to those common questions: It is important for all of the joint bone systems to have strong muscles; however, it is just as important to have flexibility, coordination, and endurance. There are many painful conditions of the back and pelvis that will not change with simple strength training, which is one of the main reasons I was compelled to write this book.

The Difference Between Strength and Coordination

Core muscles do need to be stronger in a woman who has to lift fifty pounds on a regular basis than in a woman who lifts only ten pounds. All of our muscles need to be strong enough to do all of the tasks we do day in and day out.

But the muscles of the core are constantly in use. From the moment we sit up in bed in the morning, the core is at work. That's a big difference in demand compared to the arms and the legs. Leg muscles activate when we stand and walk, then rest when we are sitting. Arm muscles are working when we reach or hold something in our hands; otherwise, they are resting. The core is active and working anytime we are upright against gravity.

These muscles are in charge of a lot of activity. We have talked quite a bit about the responsibilities of all of the functions of the core: breath, continence, organ support, and bone control. Control of the spine, pelvis, and rib cage alone is a massive responsibility. That's a lot of moving parts! We are talking about forty bones that are stacked up and held together under the load of gravity. Moreover, these bones are moving in all directions. The action of bending over to pick up a penny involves the coordination of all of these moving parts. So when discussing the core, coordination—not strength—needs to take center stage.

Strength and coordination are two very different characteristics of muscle function but are commonly misrepresented as being the same. Strength is purely about how much load a muscle can pull. Coordination is about how well a group of muscles works together to control the movement of the bones. These two qualities are measured completely differently from each other. They do share a relationship in that the more coordinated the muscles are, the better the foundation for the strength of the primary working muscle.

Training strength is simply loading the primary muscle in a certain way with exercise in order to achieve a change in how much force the primary muscle can generate. Strength is easily quantified and measured. We can measure muscle strength by moving weight or by gauging how hard the muscle can press on an object. Strength training of a muscle is not based on knowing how well the primary muscle and all of its foundational muscles are working. It's only about loading up the muscle.

There is a process to testing the strength of a muscle. Weight or some kind of resistance load is applied to the muscle in the action it performs. More pounds are added until the muscle can no longer move the weight. That max amount is the measurement used to set up a strength training program. This max amount is called the "one rep max." You know the muscle has gotten stronger with an exercise when the one rep max is increased. For example, we can measure the strength of a biceps muscle by how much it can curl. Let's say it can curl five pounds. After a structured exercise program, we can remeasure, and we know it's gotten stronger when it can curl ten pounds.

Coordination is the foundation for strength. It's the timing and speed of the muscle contraction. Moving and holding bones need the right amount of tension at the right time in the right place. A good example is the Encasement muscle's ability to hold the bones of the spine and pelvis stable. If this muscle does not have the ability to hold low tension constantly and then suddenly increase its tension when lifting, then the power of the entire lift is reduced. The Outer Core muscles cannot generate their max tension if their base of support is lost.

Coordination is measured by how well a muscle switches on and off. How fluidly can the muscle ramp up tension and ramp down? Can the muscle hold low tension for a sustained period of time? Can it adjust its holding power quickly? Just as importantly, can the muscle completely relax? It's about the quality of the muscle's contraction, paired with how well the muscle works with other muscles. Does the muscle movement flow? Is it versatile? All of these qualities are measured when testing muscle coordination.

I included this chapter in an effort to spend more time clarifying what training the control of the core should look like. There are impressions about the way things work that need to be broadened. Yes, strength is important, but coordination and muscle control are even more so. Many people take what strength training feels like and then apply those sensations to other types of exercise. In other words, they want to muscle through the exercise because they believe that's the correct way to do it.

Core Training Is Brain Training

Strength training is just loading a muscle, whereas coordination training is training the nervous system. Muscles form foundations for movement actions from muscle memory in the nervous system. Most people understand the concept of muscle memory but not necessarily how it's created. The majority of core muscle problems stem from one or more of the muscles losing their muscle memory. Muscle memory is the pattern of how muscles switch on and off in order to perform a certain movement.

Every muscle of the body has a nerve attached that fires the muscle to make it contract. If there is no nerve connected, then there is no muscle contraction. There is a nerve that contracts the muscle that comes down from the brain and hooks into the muscle. There is also a nerve that comes from the muscle and goes up into the brain to tell the brain what the muscle is actually doing.

We are born with these nerve connections from brain to muscles. All of these nerves have a specific section in the brain where they connect. These sections are mapped. The brain has a map for every nerve that goes to every muscle to make it contract. That's known as the "motor map." There is also a map for every nerve that tells the brain about what every single muscle is doing. That's called the "sensory map."

As babies, we have no muscle memories with the exception of those for breathing, sucking, and swallowing. That's all we have in our primitive brain. Infants can't even roll themselves around because the brain doesn't yet know how to make the necessary muscles work together. However, all that wiggling and squirming sends sensations of movement into the brain, and that is how memories are formed. The brain learns and encodes those lessons as memories, which build into more complicated movement patterns as we grow.

Once the brain figures out that the Breather muscle can do more than just breathe with the help of the rest of the Inner Core, it flexes, and next thing you know, you're rolling. The more the brain fires its nerve connections to the muscles, the more it feels what happens and it learns. The next thing you know, you're sitting up.

All these lessons that the brain learns about activating muscles are stored on the motor map and the sensory map. These maps interact with the memory sections of the brain, developing a veritable encyclopedia of different types of memories. This is how muscle memories are formed. This is how we can stand up from a chair and walk across the room to reach the remote control without having to think about every single muscle action. Our brain has already encoded and learned the sequencing of muscle action and reaction.

Muscle memory includes all of the actions of the different muscles that are involved with whatever movement you want to take. This includes the amount of tension in the muscle, along with the precise timing of when the muscle is supposed to kick on, then ramp tension up or down while other muscles kick into contraction. The first muscle that activates when we raise our arm is not an arm muscle, surprisingly enough. It's actually an Inner Core muscle. The body first needs a foundational support before arms or legs can move well.

Understanding how to create a new muscle memory is a big part of core training. Many of the problems women run into are either caused by a loss of muscle memory or result in the loss of muscle memory. Fortunately and unfortunately, the core muscles are very adaptable and tend to change their memory of how they are supposed to act quickly. This is a good thing when they can be restored with an investment of time and exercise. But it's a bad thing when they can change their activation process without obvious awareness.

Brain-to-Muscle Training Is Tough

I have found that one of the toughest patients to treat is another physical therapist. For one thing, it is very hard to be objective about what your body is doing. For another, when physical therapy is what you do all day long, you tend to develop strong ideas about how things should be done. Diagnosing a loss of coordination in a muscle is relatively easy when it is not in your own body. Restoring the loss of coordination in a muscle is not the same exercise progression as restoring strength to a muscle. This is difficult for everybody . . . even therapists.

Michaela was a fifty-year-old woman referred to me with significant back pain, which was starting to interfere with her practice as a physical therapist. She was mostly seeing patients with chronic back pain, so she was doing a lot of manual therapy as well as teaching exercises. She would do fairly well until about two o'clock in the afternoon, when her back pain would become so severe that she could barely rise from her stool. The painful spasms would grow progressively worse all evening until she was finally able to fall asleep, after which she'd wake up pain-free by the next morning.

Michaela's history included a pretty extensive abdominal surgery when she was sixteen. As she got older, she had several back injuries that seemed more related to overworked muscles and imbalance than to an actual trauma. She had a really tough time believing me when I told her there was a significant loss of coordination in her Encasement muscle. After all, she spent all day teaching people about core exercise and followed her own exercise routine—surely, she knew what she was doing, right? I had to fire up my real-time ultrasound imaging machine to prove to her that when she was lifting her leg or head, she was not engaging her left Encasement muscle.

It seemed reasonable to assume that this change in her Inner Core coordination had happened after her abdominal surgery, but she was not aware of any changes in her core because the muscle memory had adapted immediately. She told me that she'd always had a lot of difficulty doing sit-ups and planks. This all made perfect sense to me, because when muscle memory is lost, you have no idea that what you're feeling in your body is not "normal." You develop a new muscle memory in its place that becomes your new "normal."

The first step in restoring muscle memory is to find the muscle and reestablish a connection of awareness to that muscle with your brain. The muscle needs to become reacquainted with your brain and vice versa. Another way to think about it is to imagine that every muscle in the body is plugged into a map, which is in the brain, but the targeted muscle disconnected and needs to be plugged back into the brain. If you can't find it, you can't train it. There are tricks to finding it.

Once you can reasonably find and contract the muscle, the next step is to reestablish the ranges of tension. Muscle action is not an on-off switch. It is more like a dimmer switch. You start turning the dial of tension for a low light or low tension that can ramp up into full brightness or high tension. There are a lot of levels of tension that live in between the lowest and highest settings. The control of all these levels needs to be recovered in order to restore the Inner Core. All three of the Inner Core muscles must be able to adjust their tension levels quickly, but also be able to sustain low tension holds that fluctuate with breath. These muscles need the full spectrum of the tension dial.

One of the techniques I like to use to help my patients recover their core muscle memory is to imagine each muscle as having its own dial of tension. I guide them through the process of reestablishing a connection with the lost muscle, then I call their attention to other muscles that need to dial down. It is very common for an Outer Core muscle to ramp up its tension level in an effort to compensate for a lost muscle.

Many patients go to classes to learn about some of these core muscles, but they leave with the belief that it is best to hold the muscles as tight as possible with as much tension as possible. That's what was so challenging with my physical therapist patient, Michaela. She didn't realize that she was holding high tension in her Outer Core muscles to compensate for the loss of support from her Encasement muscle.

Practice Makes Perfect

Anytime we learn something new, we have to practice it to get good at it. This is coordination training. It's just like learning to play tennis. The swing of the racket is extremely sloppy and awkward at first, but after a while, it gets fluid and smooth and more accurate. There are five major steps to reestablishing muscle memory:

1. The first step to restoring your core coordination is believing. Sounds weird, but it's so true—if you don't believe that there's something that needs to reconnect, then the exercise just won't mean much to you. Plus, you won't do it enough.

2. Muscle memory is specific. You have to target the right muscle to do the right thing. It sounds obvious, but it's harder to pinpoint than you'd think.
3. Once you become aware of how to contract the muscle, you need to practice contracting it. Spend at least fifteen minutes every day doing a lot of repetition. More is more!
4. When the exercise becomes easy, it must be progressed and made more challenging.
5. Finally, the exercise needs to be incorporated into its functional action. In other words, the exercise of increasing the Encasement tension and strength must be practiced with bending and lifting.

It took Michaela three months before her back was feeling better. The first thing she had to do was relearn how to activate the tension of her Encasement muscle. She had such a poor connection that she could activate the Encasement muscle only when she was lying on her back. She had to practice this every day for fifteen minutes. It took her two weeks to get it down.

The next step was to activate that Encasement muscle in sitting and then in standing. That was very challenging for her because every time she tried to ramp up the tension of that muscle, she kicked up the tension of her Six-Pack and Obliques instead. The image that worked for her was to think of the dials on each muscle. She learned how to dial up tension of the Encasement but keep the Six-Pack and Obliques at the same volume.

After a month, Michaela was a master at on-off tension. So the next lesson was learning how to control the intensity as well as the duration of the tension. It took her a very long time to be able to sustain a low-level tension of the Encasement while standing and walking. Her muscle would get exhausted and then start giving out, which then gave way to the pain. This is when staying with the training gets particularly challenging for patients—when their pain persists. It seems like things should change more quickly and the pain should just go away, but that's not the reality of how the body works.

Finally, though, we got some traction on Michaela's coordination of her Encasement muscle, then she had to incorporate that tension activation back into her general core exercise program. This was harder than she thought it would be because she kept slipping back into old habits. But she stuck with it, and eventually, I'm happy to report, she's now able to work without pain!

Core Muscle Control Is Key

I have met many patients who are considered to have very good core strength, but they still have a lot of problems. These problems resolve when we're able to identify exactly what muscle is not doing what it is supposed to be doing. There's so much more to muscles than just strength, so much more they must be able to do. They must support and hold the bones wherever the bones need to go. If the muscle is too stiff from the high tension of compensating, then it doesn't matter how strong it is.

A large part of the recovery of core function relies on self-awareness. It is important to know where these muscles are located on your body in order to assess how well you are using them. This will definitively improve how effective your exercise intervention will be. Through a lifetime of movement sequencing that is recorded from the time of birth, the brain executes a series of commands to each muscle that all work together to perform all the functions necessary for successful aging. It is easy to take for granted . . . until it's gone.

When put in perspective, it is easy to see how core muscle control is part of successful aging. Again, the core is the foundation of virtually all muscle function, in that the arms and the legs rely on it as well. Arm and legs are a series of joint systems in which muscles leverage one bone and pull another bone around, much like a pulley system. The core muscles are far more complex because of their additional responsibilities.

As we age, our bodies change. The shift in hormones accompanied by changes in connective tissue results in bodies that get stiffer and a little brittle. Then there are all those other health conditions to consider. As we know, no one gets a free pass. There's always another challenge around the corner. Nevertheless, we can still live well in our bodies and feel pretty good most of the time no matter what challenges crop up.

"Motion is the lotion." "You gotta load it to grow it." These sayings hold true no matter what age you are. All of the tissues of the body are better when they are used. Fluid exchange, hydration, and nutrition for these tissues rely on movement. Using your body well and consistently makes for a much easier time aging. Keeping your brain engaged and active makes the time you have so much more enjoyable. Strength, coordination, and flexibility are the elements of resiliency, and resiliency is the ability to adjust and recover from whatever life throws at you.

PART TWO

CORE STRUGGLES AND THE PAINFUL CONSEQUENCES

CHAPTER 5

Musculoskeletal Pain

There are good and bad consequences of core exercise. Many women start an exercise routine with the intention of improving how their bodies are working. Finding the right level of intensity and the muscles to start targeting can be very difficult. There is a very aggressive attitude to exercise training these days that leads many people down the wrong road of painful consequences.

This chapter and the next explain some of the consequences of starting a core training program at the wrong level of challenge—consequences that result in more pain of the musculoskeletal body as well as in the organs that pertain to what we're calling our Lady Business.

Bad advice from the internet or, worse, inexperienced trainers/therapists/coaches lead women to believe that if the exercise isn't hard enough, then they're not doing any good. If you aren't exercising long enough or hard enough, then it's all a waste of time. This false belief contributes to inaccurate expectations from exercise, not to mention just giving up because the pain is too much to endure.

Hopefully, you are working with a good trainer/therapist/coach who understands how the core muscles work, as well as how your core muscles are working. How do you know if the exercises your trainer/therapist/coach has you doing are right for you and your body? We all expect to feel something when we exercise. Who hasn't heard "No pain, no gain" or "Pain is weakness leaving your body"? How do you know if that pain you are feeling is the right kind of pain? Read on to find out.

"No Pain, No Gain"

There is nothing more disappointing than investing time, money, and effort in something that causes you more pain and problems. This is a very common topic that comes up in my office every day. I have met numerous women who wanted to get moving by going to a Pilates or yoga class and ended up getting hurt. Another scenario is when a patient is sent to a therapist who gives them a sheet of exercises that cause not only increased pain, but also new pain in another body part they weren't having a problem with in the first place.

There are a lot of reasons why starting an exercise program can result in pain. Some of these reasons have to do with a preexisting muscle imbalance of the core muscles. Other reasons are related to compensating and cheating strategies when the exercise is too hard and you want to do it anyway. One of the most common reasons for a painful result with exercise is when the muscle becomes painful because it is already compensating for another muscle not doing its job. The exercise forces the compensating muscle to work even harder. The painful muscle is incorrectly diagnosed as being weak and given exercise to strengthen it. The end result is more pain and compensation.

The core exercises I have found to be the biggest culprits in causing more pain for women are crunches and planks. Don't get me wrong—they're both good exercises, but they are harder than expected. If you aren't using your core with the proper coordination in which all of the muscles are doing their jobs, then these exercises are not going to be effective. In fact, they will likely cause more problems.

Core Problems Cause Back Pain

There is a fairly high percentage of people walking around with some level of core muscle imbalance and limited coordination. That doesn't mean that these people are necessarily suffering with back pain. It really depends on their lifestyle. If you spend most of your day in front of a computer and then go home and eat, watch TV, and go to bed, then there isn't a lot of physical challenge in your lifestyle. The body can harbor all kinds of stiffnesses and compensation without actually causing pain.

An unfortunate truth is that this type of lifestyle leads to deconditioning and all kinds of health issues. That makes for a situation that doesn't age well. In order to feel pretty good in those golden years, you really want to keep your muscles in working condition as well as maintain some level of good cardiovascular fitness. How you feel is really dependent on how healthy your physical body is.

Core muscle problems can cause different kinds of pain and dysfunction for the different parts of the body. This chapter focuses on why muscle imbalances cause musculoskeletal pain. Most researchers and pain experts agree that a common source of pain is either too much stress tension or too much compression pressure applied to tissue of the musculoskeletal body. This also holds true for visceral tissues (further explained in the next chapter).

The parts of the musculoskeletal body most commonly impacted by a core problem include the upper back, the low back, the pelvis, and the hips. The spine is really just a big stack of bones that has an extensive collection of *ligaments*—gristly bits that connect and hold the bones together. There are also gristly bits that live in between the bones for the purposes of cushioning movement, and these include the discs and cartilage that line the joints.

Researchers have done a lot of experiments on the bones and gristly connective tissues of the spine because it is important to understand just how strong these gristly bits are and how much they can be relied on to support their bones. These studies discovered that when you carve away all the muscles of the spine and then put a load of weight on the bones, those gristly bits do not hold up very well under the pressure of weight. In fact, the stack of bones starts to buckle and bend at just under twenty pounds of pressure, which is far less than the weight of the body itself.

This buckling under twenty pounds demonstrates just how important the core muscle system is to the health of the bones of the spine, the rib cage, and the pelvis, as well as all of their associated gristly bits. When the core muscles are not able to hold and control the bones well, then more strain of the load has to be carried through the connective tissues. This is what breaks down first with little microtears. When you accumulate enough microtears, then you get inflammation. Tears and inflammation cause pain. When we get pain, it's a normal response to tense up that part of the body to protect it. This protective guarding just causes more inflammation and pain. It's a vicious cycle that's tough to break.

Another common scenario that leads to the vicious cycle is when the core muscles are too stiff. This is common because it's related to the typical sedentary lifestyle of sitting a lot. When you sit for more than 75 percent of your day, the body responds to that. Backs, hips, and hamstrings get tight, and then things don't work well mechanically and become painful. The spine and cage have a lot of moving parts that have to slide and glide. A stiff muscle group will limit that slide and glide. A stiff, tight muscle will add an extra squeeze and compression to the bone. This results in pinching or getting stuck.

The Pain of Compensation

Where things can really get complicated is in understanding that pain can be the consequence of both things happening—in other words, when one muscle is too weak to do its job, so then another muscle has to compensate by ramping up its tension and working harder. This compensating muscle gets stiff and tight. A stiff, tight muscle pinches and compresses. Both muscle problems can cause different pain for different reasons. Neither the pain related to this nor the root problem itself will go away until both causes—the weakness and the tightness—are corrected.

This is the heart of what I do for a living. My specialty as a physical therapist is chronic pain, and the most challenging patients are those suffering with back pain. Getting to the source of where that pain is coming from is the true challenge.

There are a lot of women who struggle with back pain related to core muscle imbalances. While I have heard many different stories, there's one in particular that really represents some of the difficulties certain women go through. When I met Letty, she was sixty-three years old. She told me that she'd never had any problems with her back until she delivered her second child, many years ago. She just assumed that back problems came with the territory of bearing children and that they weren't really relevant to her current pain problem.

I asked her the usual questions about pain during her pregnancy and postpartum period, but her answers didn't really correlate with the kind of pain she was having now. She told me she'd been living with a constant low-grade ache over the right side of her low back, which actually started a year after her delivery. But that wasn't the pain that brought her to physical therapy. The actual pain that brought her to my office was extremely severe when she would twist her body, and it was very localized to the right lower side of her rib cage.

Letty had been seeing a chiropractor for years in order to help with her lower-back pain. She told me that the chiropractic treatment always gave her relief, but the pain would just keep coming back. Around ten years ago, this back pain became more constant, which led her to try other things like massage therapy and acupuncture. For a while, the massage really seemed to help and she was managing pretty well in her life.

A year before she met me, Letty's daughter talked her into trying a Pilates class. Letty had been told over and over that core strengthening would be good for her back, so she agreed. Plus, Letty really wanted to support her daughter, who had gained a significant amount of weight. She said her daughter had always struggled with her weight and this was the first time she was excited about any kind of exercise.

So Letty started taking these classes with her daughter, but she wasn't impressed. Everything was hard to do. Everything felt heavy and sweaty, and she was always breathing harder than everyone else in class. It was embarrassing because she was not the oldest one there. Not even close! There were a few seventy-year-olds who were kicking her butt. Between wanting to keep up with the overachievers and trying to set a good example for her daughter, Letty kept going . . . but it never got any easier.

She finally stopped going when she woke up one morning and couldn't get out of bed because of a new pain. A twisting, stabbing pain in her side that got worse when she moved. At first, she told me, she was kind of happy about this pain because it gave her a good excuse to skip Pilates class. But then this pain didn't go away. In fact, it just got worse.

When she went to her doctor about it, she was sent out for all kinds of tests. She told me all of these tests ended up costing her close to ten thousand dollars. But still she had no answers after all that testing, time, and money. So her doctor decided she must be having a muscle problem and referred her for physical therapy.

After getting her full history of the different types of pain, it was time for me to assess how her body was working. The first thing I noticed was her posture. She had a very pronounced arch in her back. Her cage was aimed high and her pelvis was tipped down. Her most intense pain was very localized to the lower ribs in the front, where the ribs become a thick cartilage. This is also the place where the Obliques and the Six-Pack attach. It was easy to see that her ribs were jammed up and the muscles were inflamed. The challenge was figuring out why she got like this from Pilates.

We therefore delved into looking at her core muscle control. There was no activation of the Encasement muscle on the right at all. In fact, the appearance of the abdomen was very rounded, protruding on the right but more curved at the waistline on the left. She also had terrible breath mechanics. When she would inhale deeply, only her chest would lift—a clear sign that she was not using her Breather muscle the right way.

Letty's story started to come together. It was obvious to me that her posture had been affected by her pregnancy. Women have to change their posture to make space for a growing baby. That posture doesn't just revert back after having the baby. When the posture changes like this, it affects how the muscles of the Inner Core line up. The Breather muscle plate is tipped and can't work effectively, so Letty was getting very short of breath with exercise, which can contribute to jamming up the ribs. The Encasement muscle can't activate well when the posture of the other muscle plates is not well aligned.

Letty's original pain was due to the lack of Encasement support on the right side, which was probably caused by having a baby. The Encasement muscle has a tough time recovering from pregnancy and many times never recovers its full capacity of control. The core then compensates by using the Outer Core muscles to fill in for the weakness of the Encasement. Letty's second, more severe pain came from trying to force an exercise program that was too hard on a body that was not coordinated and balanced.

The loss of connection and support on one side of the spine causes more stress and strain on the gristly ligaments and connective tissues. When the bones lose their support in movement and holding, then the strain is placed on the gristle that holds the bones together. Over time, the gristle experiences microtearing, which then becomes inflammatory. That can cause that low-grade, dull ache.

When Letty got going with core strengthening exercises, the second pain came in. The Oblique muscles attach to the areas of the ribs where Letty's pain was. These Oblique muscles were already overworking, trying to hold things together. Adding more exercise stress caused a big overload on the parts of the muscles where they turn into gristly tendon to attach to the bone. Letty's exercise had caused her to develop tendonitis.

When I explained to Letty that the pain she was having was the result of a muscle imbalance of the Inner Core, with one side of the Encasement being very weak and her Breather muscle not working well, she was confused. How could that be? she asked. Nobody had ever told her she had a breathing problem. How can breath cause pain? I had to explain to her how Pressure Mechanics works as well as how muscles compensate. Once she understood that the exercises she was doing are not the kind that will help with this sort of weakness, she was able to change her core control. She was even able to return to Pilates after recovering her core function and changing her posture.

This story is not only a great example of how a life event can change the inner workings of the body and Pressure Mechanics. Letty's case also shows how these types of changes can cause more trouble as we age depending on what we are doing. It is easy to focus therapy intervention only on where the pain is. The key to recovery is to take into account how the entire system is working and piece together all of the life events and their contribution to how this system is working. The common line of thinking is that problems that result from life events will just go away. And, in fact, the pain and problems associated with pregnancy often do go away. But you can't assume that the body will just naturally restore itself.

I have seen many women who "try to get their core back" with a core program. They are correct in believing that there is something not working properly; they just don't know what it is. Most of these women are so discouraged from developing new pains or never seeing any improvement that they just give up. The sad truth is that their condition just continues to deteriorate as they age.

So How Do You Know What's Going On?

There are as many types of painful compensations as there are muscles in the body, and many of them are not painful. So how do you know when the exercise that you are trying is okay for you? It is true that certain types of soreness are natural when you first start a new exercise program. Most of us can remember that time when we went the extra mile and paid the price for it the next day.

Training soreness has to do with starting a new activity or increasing the challenge of a current activity. This soreness is generally caused by *lactic acid*, a by-product of the muscles' use of energy. And this type of pain has its own name: DOMS, or delayed onset muscle soreness. It comes on later, after the exercise, and resolves itself within a day or two. If you are experiencing DOMS after every single exercise session, then the pain is likely not related to just the newness of the activity. You are either exercising too aggressively for muscle metabolism or overloading some gristly bit of your body and causing inflammation.

If you start feeling pain in a part of the body in which you've never felt before, then you should stop what you are doing and ask a professional about it. A good trainer/therapist/coach will want to know about that and should be able to problem-solve it. There are adjustments to technique or challenges that should be made. You shouldn't feel like your concern means you can't handle being challenged or that you're trying to get out of doing something difficult.

The best strategy for ensuring success when embarking on a new routine is to educate yourself. It is extremely important to have a working knowledge of how your parts operate in general. It is also important to know what to expect. Significant pain during or immediately after exercise is not okay. Pain in a different part of your body that doesn't go away is not okay. If your trainer/therapist/coach doesn't really know why you're in pain or doesn't offer options for changing something about your program, then it's time to seek advice elsewhere.

Never give up on yourself. There is always an answer, even if it doesn't seem relevant. Our bodies are made of cells, and cells can always grow and adapt in a healthy way. We are never too old or too broken for exercise intervention. Everyone has the capacity to get better.

CHAPTER 6

Organ Consequences

"The 'Top Twenty Core Exercises' program I got off the internet has caused me to leak. How is that possible?" . . . "My Pilates class seems to have something to do with my constipation? How can that happen?" These are questions I hear about the unexpected and unwanted consequences of core exercise, and they point to precisely why it is extremely important to start any core program at the right level of challenge with the right technique.

It is hard to comprehend the complexity of the core muscles. Many people are surprised when they learn that Inner Core muscle tension can have an effect on digestion and circulation. How can a muscle influence how well the colon does its job? It is very common for people to question why doing a breath exercise is helpful. Why do problems with breath contribute to organ prolapse? Why are young women developing problems with continence when they've never had a baby?

There is a surprisingly strong relationship between the Inner Core and the organ system. When I talk about the "organ system," I am including everything between the Breather muscle and the Floor. This includes the liver and stomach at the top, the small bowel, kidneys, and colon in the middle, and the bladder, uterus, and rectum at the bottom, as well as the entire circulatory system.

That is a lot of blood, guts, and air. As explained in chapter 3, I group all of these organs and blood vessels into what I like to visualize as an internal water balloon. This water balloon is sandwiched between the Breather muscle at the top and the Floor muscle at the bottom. The action of the Floor and Breather is much like an elastic plate that contracts to flatten or expand and lengthens into bowl shapes. This balloon sandwich is connected all the way around by the Encasement muscle.

Quick Review of the Jobs of the Outer Core and the Inner Core

The Inner Core muscles do not move the bones; however, they do move the organ system. The movement of the organ system is breath. This is the action that is not well understood or envisioned. There are numerous health benefits of breath and breath exercise, but it is hard to imagine how just taking a deep breath does all that—moves the entire organ system. Oxygen is great, but how does it help with constipation or continence?

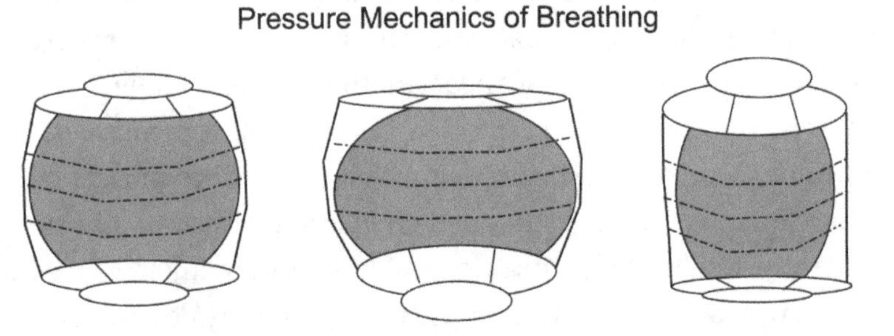

This is what breath looks like using the internal water balloon model. When the Breather muscle contracts, it flattens and expands in order to draw air into the lungs. When the Breather muscle flattens and expands, it pushes downward on the water balloon.

The Encasement muscle also expands with the Breather muscle as it inhales air. Its expansion supports the water balloon as it is pressed downward by the Breather. Recall that the organ balloon moves as much as two centimeters during breath action. The Floor muscle deepens and lengthens to cup and support the organs during inhalation.

As air is exhaled from the lungs, the Breather muscle needs to return to its bowl-shaped plate. The Encasement and the Floor also return to their start positions. When air is slowed down or resisted leaving the body, the Encasement and the Floor contract with more force to push the air out. This is also the basis for singing and talking.

So there is up-and-down movement of the water balloon as well as expansion. The organs within this balloon love this motion. Breathing is kind of like an internal massage for the organ system.

The colon and small bowel love the massage movement of breath. They have a lot of work to do moving and digesting food. There are many twists and turns through which the by-products of digestion must navigate. The action of breathing churns the intestines and helps keep things moving along.

The circulatory system also loves the breath action of the Inner Core. This system consists of vessels that carry oxygenated blood to the far reaches of the body, but that blood needs to return back to the heart and lungs for an O_2 fill-up. The action of breath has been described as a sump pump for circulation. It helps move the blood back up the body.

Once you see just how these Inner Core muscles are moving and interacting with the balloon of organs, it is easier to understand how important the tension levels are. Each muscle of the Inner Core has a certain range of tension that is needed to perform the action of breath.

This tension level will ramp up depending on the amount of support the bones need. The tension levels of these muscles will be higher while breathing and moving a heavy package, but lower when just breathing and walking. Problems start developing if the tension levels get out of sync.

The Inner Core and Digestion

Alycia was a really pleasant twenty-two-year-old who was sent to me for chronic neck pain. Her pain was a musculoskeletal consequence of her out-of-control core, but she had organ consequences as well.

Alycia was the poster child for exercise and nutrition. She was extremely diligent in managing her food choices, not because she was concerned about her weight, but because she had terrible constipation.

She was aware of the dangers of relying on laxatives (not to mention the embarrassment), so she was very careful about her diet. She also went to the gym every day and did an hour of weight training. She was told this would help her constipation.

The reason for her neck pain was the same reason for her digestion trouble. She had *kyphosis*, a type of scoliosis characterized more by a forward curve of the upper back and rib cage than by a tip to the side. Kyphosis is the enemy posture of women everywhere, resulting in that typical slumped-looking posture that resembles a turtle shell. Being slumped part of the time is not really that big a deal. It becomes a big deal when we stay in that posture all of the time. It becomes an even bigger deal if we get really stiff and can't move out of the posture and straighten up.

When we slump forward in kyphosis, the top-plate Breather muscle becomes pressurized on top of the organ water balloon. This constant push from the Breather muscle puts a downward pressure on the organs. That's okay . . . until it isn't. This pressure needs to let up from time to time.

To help us understand, here's a quick review of Pressure Mechanics and posture:

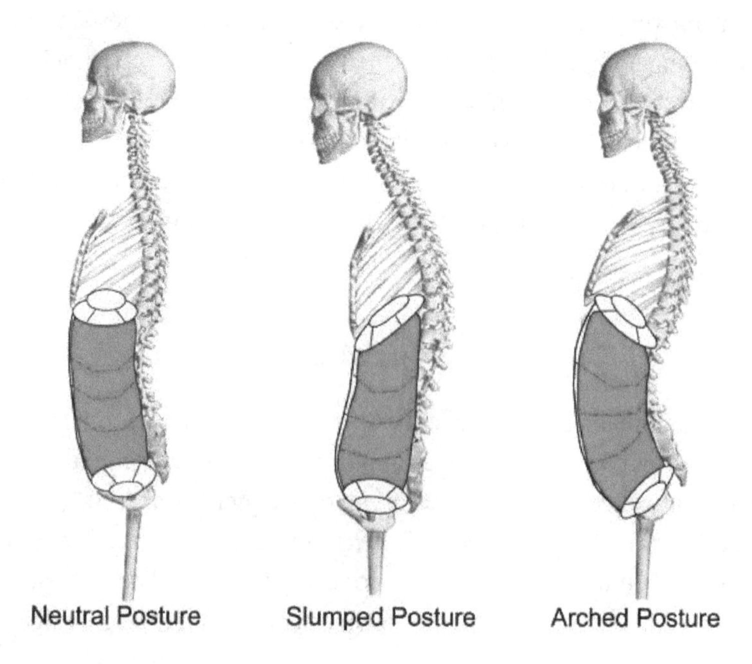

Alycia was very consistent with her exercise, which would make her the dream patient of any physical therapist, right? Unfortunately, Alycia wasn't doing her exercises with good technique. She met a young trainer at the gym who taught her to just power through all of her core exercises. She was able to get through most of them by holding her breath to cheat. When she was not allowed to hold her breath, she was very disappointed to discover that she was very weak and couldn't do most of them.

So, when you consider the effects of the forward slump of Alycia's posture causing pressure on the water balloon, paired with overworking her breath holds, the picture starts to fill in. She had no flattening or expansion to her inhalation and even less length to her exhalation. Her colon was under a constant state of compression with little to no assistance from breath action.

It took quite a bit of conversation to persuade Alycia to put her core exercises on hold while we loosened up her upper-back rib cage. Basically, she had to relearn how to breathe. She needed quite a bit of coordination training with this because she had no real muscle memory of what good breath felt like. Then she needed coordination training for how to properly use all of her core muscles.

Alycia was a great success story not only because her neck pain improved significantly, but also because she was able to resolve the majority of her constipation problems. She was told that it was unlikely that her condition would ever improve because her scoliosis was just a part of her genetics and could not be changed. Though it's true that a curvature of the spine cannot be removed, it is possible—and extremely important—to make that curve as flexible and coordinated as possible.

Inner Core and Continence / Organ Prolapse

The profession of physical therapy is based on what science tells us about how the body works. The good news is that we are always learning. The bad news is that it takes a while for science to catch up with all the different aspects of how the body works. I graduated from physical therapy school thirty years ago. What we did in physical therapy was a little different than what we do now, informed by the advancements of the past decade or two. I had always assumed that when women had trouble with continence, that automatically meant their Floor muscles were weak. Whereas this is true in some cases, it is not in others.

The Floor muscles support the entire organ water balloon and are directly supportive of the bladder, uterus, and colon. The Floor hosts the urethra, the vagina, and the anus—the organ passages to the outside. The Floor needs to have sufficient strength and endurance to maintain closure of these sphincters to manage the storage of excrement. In other words, a good, strong Floor needs to hold the pee and the poo until it's time.

A really important core truth is that the Floor can be strong but still have a problem with continence. This is where the relationship among the Inner Core muscles can cause trouble. The scenario is similar to the story of Alycia, in that it involves a woman having problems with breath holding habits and bad posture. Alycias' breath and posture were creating a lot of downward pressure on her organ system (water balloon) and contributing to constipation. These mechanics can also contribute to incontinence. This pressure can interfere with digestion, but it can also load the bladder, uterus, and colon so heavily that the Floor gives out. The Floor muscles can be well coordinated and strong enough to do their job but still give out under pressure that is higher than they are engineered to manage.

A woman with this kind of pressure system could do Pelvic Floor exercises all day long but never improve her continence. That is the frustration for many women—doing an exercise that is supposed to be good for you but never actually helps the problem. Unfortunately, it doesn't just end with occasional issues with incontinence. It becomes progressively worse with age. As we get older, there are changes in how well things hold related to drops in available estrogen. After menopause, everything seems to drop. This is the common explanation for organ prolapse. It has to do with the strength of the connective tissue as well as the flexibility. The stiffer and more rigid, the less resiliency, the less slide and glide. The less support in the face of pressure.

Organ prolapse is when the bladder, uterus, or rectum fall in on one another and then out through the Floor. There are a variety of very effective surgeries that will string the organ back up and support the

Floor—that's the upside. The flip side is that up to 50 percent of these surgeries fail after three to five years. A huge percentage of women need two, sometimes three surgeries for this same issue in their lifetime. Many women just don't want to go through it again, so they put up with the discomfort of prolapse.

Given how good the surgical options are, it doesn't seem to make sense that there isn't something more that can prevent prolapse from happening again. There is, actually—and once again, it involves the habits of posture and breath. It *is* possible to change how the organ water balloon is pressurized. We'll cover these issues more thoroughly in chapter 8, but for now I want to drive home the point that incontinence is not something that women should just sit back and accept.

Leaking Is Not Just a Part of Life

It is remarkable how many online videos I have come across showing young women lifting amazingly high amounts of weight over their head while peeing themselves. Although it's a fine thing to be strong enough to get that far with lifting, I don't see this as truly mastering the task. Something is giving out.

The bigger concern I have about this is the message it sends to other young women—that involuntarily urinating in the midst of performing a favored activity is okay. It's certainly nothing to be ashamed of; it happens under certain conditions, but it is a sign that you should get some help. If you are leaking, then you should talk to a specialist or get an opinion from someone trained in this area.

Anytime you start or accelerate an exercise program and leaking starts to happen, you should find out what's going on with your Inner Core and your Pressure Mechanics. This doesn't mean you should never repeat the new exercise; it means there is something going on that could be improved upon.

This is particularly important for women to understand as they age. Starting to leak at a young age *does* contribute to more problems later. It's been assumed that a certain amount of incontinence is just part of the life of a woman, but that's just not true. I cannot say this often enough. It is essential for women to be aware of how their core muscles are working. Life events can cause changes in the Pressure Mechanics, as well as in how the muscles are coordinating. Imagine having a surgery for prolapse but never restoring how the muscles work. This is extremely common. Then imagine the consequences of joining a core exercise class or trying the "Top Twenty Core Exercises" regimen!

I have found that the first step to successful rehab is restoring the coordination of and muscle memory to all the muscles of the core. Educating women is critical. While it can be very time-consuming to find the right expert and then retrain all your muscle memories, it is a very worthwhile investment of your time and energy. You will thank yourself thirty years from now!

CHAPTER 7

Pregnancy

Now we transition to different health conditions that affect women more commonly than men. These health conditions cause specific changes in how the Inner Core muscles work with consequences on the Pressure Mechanics. It helps to understand what these health conditions are, as well as how they impact muscle function of the core.

I was surprised to discover what a challenge estrogen can be for our bodies. This hormone affects the health of a lot of different organ systems. Estrogen is one of those things that is tough to live with and tougher to live without. It's tough to be a lady!

It is all too common to see women hope for the best in terms of getting their bodies back after giving birth. Many diet themselves into a corner because they can't get rid of that pooch. The pooch really has nothing to do with weight but, rather, with a loss of Encasement muscle memory. The struggle is real, but dieting won't change it. Nor will an aggressive core training program that starts with the top ten ways to plank.

Continence and organ prolapse are serious health conditions for women. One of the main reasons for admittance to a nursing home is incontinence. Many health care workers around the world, myself included, wonder what that statistic would look like if women knew that more could be done for their health. It's also interesting how lung and gut problems, too, fall victim to pressure and contribute to incontinence and prolapse.

Osteoporosis and back pain drive many women to try an exercise routine for their health. I see patients every day after they've tried a new program and developed a new problem as a result. It would be wonderful to have more information about the core available for everyone in an effort to prevent that from happening. I want to work myself out of a job.

The Profound Changes of Pregnancy

Pregnancy is a women-only health condition that profoundly changes the body and core. While having a baby is a blessing, the process of growing the baby can be challenging for our bodies. Babies occupy space, and we must expand and change the function of every single core muscle we have to accommodate this process. Having a baby is one of the most common reasons that many women get involved with a core program. They want to get their bodies back!

It is extremely important to understand how the changes in the Inner Core impact the pressure system. I cannot stress this strongly enough. There is a lot of focus on the abdominal wall and the Pelvic Floor for obvious reasons, but it's crucial to remember that the Breather muscle changes too. Not breathing well can create huge problems when jumping into a core program.

There are also a lot of women who, for a variety of reasons, never had the time to restore their core after having a baby. Those first six months are exhausting! New mothers are sleep deprived and struggling with so many demands on their bodies. That first year is so draining, and there is very little time for self-care. In fact, you're lucky to get a shower most days! Unfortunately, the changes in the physical body remain, and so there's always the potential for some women to go on to develop pain and organ trouble as they age due to the Inner Core changes caused by pregnancy.

Core Changes Throughout Pregnancy

Changes in a woman's physical body begin earlier in pregnancy than you might think. The first trimester involves a large shift in the hormones estrogen and progesterone, as well as in a bunch of other types of hormonal activity. This is the body's way of setting the stage for preparing to accommodate a growing fetus.

The changes in how we breathe can start as early as the first trimester. Hormonal shifts in estrogen and progesterone actually begin to change how the airway passages work in the lungs this early. We get nauseous, tired, and constipated. Plus, we have to pee more . . . even in the first trimester. All because of hormones!

During the second trimester, the reason for all of these hormonal shifts begins to make itself known. The baby is growing! The Breather muscle starts to stiffen and lose its downward excursion, and the Encasement muscle is lengthening. Changes in our bony structure start to happen. The rib cage begins to expand along with the pelvis. Ligament—that gristly connective tissue that holds our bones together—becomes lax so that the cage and pelvis can expand.

It is also during the second trimester when women might start to see signs of the dreaded *diastasis* of the Rectus Abdominis, which is when the connective tissue that holds the Six-Pack together starts to develop some laxity and stretch open. This is part of the spreading of the abdominal wall. This connective tissue or gristly fascia, otherwise known as the aponeurosis, you may recall, is that white section in the center of the abdominal wall that connects the right and left muscles of the Encasement and the Obliques. This connective tissue envelops the Six-Pack on each side. The connective tissue from all these layers meets in the middle, in between the Six-Pack, and is called the *linea alba*.

As the hormones elevate, they cause a laxity or loosening of this linea alba in order to make the entire abdominal wall more pliable to stretching and lengthening for the baby. Some studies report that these kinds of changes can start as early as fourteen weeks. It is really important to keep in mind that everyone is different in terms of how all this can happen.

By the time you reach the third trimester, the baby is really taking up space. The rib cage and pelvis are literally rocked back, throwing the spine into a lot of extension to make room for the baby. The stomach, liver, and majority of the intestines are under a lot of pressure because the baby is crowding them up under the Breather muscle. The bladder and rectum are also suffering from the pressure of being under the growing baby.

It is during this final trimester that the Encasement and other abdominal muscles have to really stretch and lengthen to accommodate the baby. Studies show that at thirty-five weeks of pregnancy, almost 100 percent of women are likely to have a diastasis. Keep in mind that this is a normal part of being pregnant. Many women worry a lot about that and want to prevent it. Although there are certain risk factors that can cause the diastasis to become quite wide, the extent of the diastasis has more to do with how many babies you've had and how well you're able to recover the strength and control of your core in between babies.

Importantly, the posture of a pregnant woman's body changes in the last trimester. The cage is thrown back as women start to lead with their bellies. This change in the cage really affects how the Diaphragm muscle works. To use the Pressure Mechanics model, the Breather plate and the Floor muscle plate totally change their orientation with the water balloon while the Encasement expands.

These changes don't necessarily reverse themselves after pregnancy. Many women continue to have a lot of arch in their back, with their Breather muscle tipped up and their Floor tipped down. The ligaments that hold the bones together have endured a lot of change as well during this process, and this doesn't just revert either once the baby is no longer there.

All of the stiffening that occurs might need to be addressed and mobilized for the woman to recover her natural posture. This is relevant to the Breather and Floor muscles as well: They have to go where the posture puts them, so they are particularly dependent on the posture of their bony homes. This means that the Breather muscle has changed how it loads the water balloon of pressure, and the Floor has changed how it supports the water balloon of pressure.

These changes in the core also affect the hip muscles. Pregnant women late in their third trimester tend to start swaying quite a bit as they walk. The hip muscles can't work the same because the belly load is so different and the pelvis is more tipped. That changes how the hip muscles work. This is another thing to consider once the baby is delivered: how to get your butt back. The hip muscles carry the core around, and they depend on the alignment of the pelvic base of the core. They get weaker and stiffer as the pelvic base changes.

What's the First Thing You Can Do?

So where do new moms begin with regaining control of their physical bodies right after giving birth? That is a really tough question to answer accurately because there are so many different ways women's bodies change. Much of it has to do with whether or not you had a vaginal delivery or a C-section. Did you develop a diastasis? Were there any complications during the pregnancy or delivery? What was your fitness level prior to getting pregnant?

The first resource is your obstetrician. Your OB-GYN will provide you with guidelines on what is safe to begin and when. Once you get the green light from your doctor to resume certain activities, it's time to start prioritizing self-care; however, keep in mind that your body has been through a lot in a relatively short period of time.

Most physicians advise postpartum moms to be gentle with their bodies for the first six to eight weeks after delivery. This is the amount of time it takes just for the genitourinary organs to recover. It is normal to feel a lot of weakness and pain in your back and bottom, as well as a tendency to leak or an inability to control gas. If you are still experiencing these symptoms after eight weeks, then it is important to consult with your doctor and a therapist before doing anything more physical.

There is a lot of change in the muscles and ligaments of the rib cage, spine, and pelvis during pregnancy. Think about how much expansion and hormonal shifting happened within a nine-month period. You also need to remember that those hormonal changes are still present and that it takes a while for all of those changes to settle down. In fact, it can take up to six months for these tissues and muscles to recover before they can tolerate the load of strengthening.

This is extremely important for new moms and core muscle recovery. Resist the desire to rush into the gym. Start with breathing. At the end of the book, there is a little self-assessment that walks you through how to check your breathing and how to reacquaint yourself with your Floor and Encasement muscles. Breath work is core work. You want to get that Diaphragm mobilized.

It is also important to think about where you are in your posture, but be very cautious with the struggle. Again, it takes a bit of time for everything to settle back down and for all those tissues to restabilize. Awareness is helpful, but don't bully your tissues.

The disruption to and lack of quality sleep is a big deal not only for how you feel in general, but also for how your tissues are recovering. Too many women are used to multitasking their way through. They end up exceeding what their physical body is capable of, then feel unsuccessful. These tissues and muscles are going to feel fatigued a lot quicker than they used to. They will recover, though!

Key Considerations Specific to Pregnancy and Core Recovery

There are a few key issues associated with pregnancy and the core that are worth mentioning: diastasis recovery, incontinence, and pelvic organ prolapse. Here's an overview of what we actually know about each of these issues based on the current research.

Diastasis

As I said earlier, studies report that almost 100 percent of women have a diastasis by thirty-five weeks of pregnancy. Of these women, 40 percent still had a diastasis at six months postpartum. Some women never fully recover and resolve their diastasis. There is a lot of concern among pregnant mothers because nobody wants to have a doming protrusion in the middle of their belly, and it would be nice to know how to prevent it.

Many studies have been done to identify the risk factors for having a diastasis that never resolves. Interestingly enough, they did not find any meaningful association with the amount of weight gained during pregnancy nor the amount a woman weighed before getting pregnant. There wasn't any statistical significance associated with the baby's weight, either. There was some evidence that the number of pregnancies was a contributing factor, however, as well as how well core strength and endurance was recovered in between each pregnancy.

The good news is that many women can recover. There are plenty of studies that show a good core exercise program can help reduce the diastasis. The interesting thing is that it really needs to be an all-inclusive program, though. In other words, you can't just plank your way through this. The alignment of the cage and pelvis needs to be restored. Good breath and Pressure Mechanics must be regained. A diastasis cannot be restored unless these issues have been addressed.

No woman is the same as any other, much like no pregnancy is the same, so obviously, recovery depends on the severity of the diastasis. Some women do require surgery to correct it because the diastasis is just too wide. These ladies also need to follow up with the same process of recovering their core mechanics. Surgery is not a quick fix for the abdominal wall. All muscles still have to be recoordinated and connected.

Incontinence

It is somewhat amusing to see all of the Mother's Day memes that reference incontinence as a part of a woman's fate, but it's simply not true for everyone. While quite a few women become incontinent after pregnancy, that doesn't mean they are doomed to be so forever. Almost half of first-time pregnant women have some leakage during their third trimester, and three-fourths of women who have multiple babies experience leakage. Unfortunately, about 50 percent of all women who have given birth report ongoing leakage issues five years later.

The main reason for these high numbers has to do with the lack of core recovery. It is hard to understand that the core as a whole needs to be recovered, not just the Floor. Many women can have perfectly good Floor strength, but their Pressure Mechanics can remain altered with too much pressure on the Floor. All of that pressure can cause the Floor to get tired and give way to leakage.

Pelvic Organ Prolapse

Pelvic organ prolapse is when the organs at the bottom of the water balloon collapse and droop in on one another and then down and out. The organs involved include the bladder, the uterus, the vagina, the rectum, and sometimes the small bowel. These organs are subjected to all of the pressures from above and really rely on the slings of muscle and connective tissue of the Floor.

The official term *cele* refers to a bulging of a pelvic organ into the wall of the vagina. A *cystocele* is when the bladder droops over onto the vagina. If the vaginal wall is weak enough, the bladder and sometimes the urethra can drop down and out of the vagina. A *rectocele* is when the rectum collapses into the back wall of the vagina. All of these conditions can be painful and cause incontinence.

There are a lot of reasons why pelvic organ prolapse develops, and pregnancy is a major one. Sometimes delivering the baby will just cause too much damage to the connective tissue of the Floor and vagina. Most of the time, the problem really has more to do with too much pressure rather than actual damage. The kyphotic postures have shown a very high contribution to women developing pelvic organ prolapse because these postures put a lot of load onto the pressure system.

Numerous types of surgery target pelvic organ prolapse. It's not really useful to describe the specific surgeries here because they're continually evolving and vary in their effectiveness, but the unfortunate truth is that most of these surgeries fail. Some studies claim that as much as 50 percent of these surgeries fail. A huge reason for that is that the source of the prolapse—why it occurred—has not been addressed. It is extremely important to restore the core and posture for the health of the Floor.

Core Recovery

Obviously, there are a lot of really good reasons for investing time and energy in a comprehensive core program after having a baby. It truly makes a difference in how comfortable we can be in our bodies as we get older. Incontinence is one of the primary reasons for admittance to a nursing home assisted living and for the high cost of care for women.

A good place to start in your own recovery process is the self-assessment tool and collection of Inner Core exercises you'll find in the last part of this book. There are a lot of good programs available that seem to be evolving all of the time. The most important and valuable thing you can do for your health is to understand your body's mechanics. If you are peeing or pooping when you don't mean to, then you must seek professional help. If you are hurting or not breathing well while moving, working, or exercising, then you must stop and seek professional help. If you understand your Pressure Mechanics and these basic concepts, then you will know if the trainer, therapist, or any other provider you are working with is actually helping you or not.

CHAPTER 8

Incontinence and Pelvic Organ Prolapse

After a chapter on how pregnancy changes the core, the two topics of incontinence and pelvic organ prolapse are ideal to discuss next. Although we did touch on these subjects in the previous chapter, there is more to understand.

Almost all the women I have talked to about these issues believe that incontinence and organ prolapse are inevitable outcomes of pregnancy and aging. They believe that when you have babies, you will become incontinent. If you didn't become incontinent at that point, then you will when you grow older and go through menopause. If you are leaking after a baby, then you will probably have a prolapse after menopause.

It is understandable that women come away with these beliefs considering what our bodies go through to grow and deliver a baby. But when you start really sifting through the research of the last ten years, you start to understand that there's actually a lot more to this story. This truly is the kind of knowledge that should be available to all women about how their bodies work because it has a big impact on how comfortable we are in our bodies as we live our lives and on how successfully we will age.

Incontinence Defined

The majority of information sources agree that there are three kinds of incontinence, while other sources talk about five. We will focus on the top three because they are the most pertinent to what women commonly experience.

1. Stress Incontinence

Stress incontinence occurs when the pressure inside and/or outside the bladder exceeds the ability of the Pelvic Floor muscles to support and hold closed the urethra, the tube from the bladder that allows urine to pass. The main point here is that the pressure overcomes the Pelvic Floor muscles' ability to hold the pee. There are a couple of different situations in which this happens, both of which are important to understand because the different problems have different solutions.

- If the muscles of the Pelvic Floor are truly weak, then the normal pressures within a bladder that is filling with urine will not be well supported. This weakness will cause leaking even with a normal volume of urine in the bladder.
- If there is a lot of pressure on the outside of the bladder, such as high tension of the Breather muscle, there will be leaking accidents because constant tension causes constant pressure on the bladder, which will overload the Pelvic Floor muscles. Once the muscles become overwhelmed, they cannot support the urethra and then leakage occurs.

Then there are those moments of extra pressure. Activities that cause extra pressure on the bladder can become sources of potential embarrassment. These activities include laughing, coughing, and sneezing. During these activities, the Diaphragm pushes down on the pressure system with sudden bursts of high-intensity tension. If the Pelvic Floor muscles are weak, then they won't be able to hold against the sudden increase in pressure. If there is already a lot of pressure from the Breather muscle pushing on the system, then adding more pressure will overwhelm the Pelvic Floor muscles.

Other activities also cause increased pressure on the bladder system, like running, jumping, and lifting. These activities can become so problematic that women eventually avoid them. Running and jumping produce a lot of jarring forces that the body has to absorb. The multitasking Floor muscles have so many jobs to do at once! They need to hold constant low tension to support the pelvis and the organ pressure. It also needs to contract quickly with bursts of higher tension for the extra pounding pressure of running and jumping.

Lifting heavy weights generates extremely high pressure on the system. Strength training exercises really require the entire Inner Core system to work well. The Breather muscle needs to be moving well through its full excursion with the right level of connection support from its Encasement muscle, and the Floor needs to have the right level of strength and coordination to support the system and the dynamics of breath.

2. Urge Incontinence

The second kind of incontinence is known as *urge incontinence*—when you really don't think you need to use the bathroom that bad until you get near a bathroom. Once your brain registers that there is a bathroom nearby, it tells the bladder, which suddenly decides that not only it is time to go, but it must do so immediately.

Urge incontinence is different than stress incontinence because it involves just the structure of the bladder rather than the entire system in which the bladder is living. The bladder has its very own muscle in its walls called the *detrusor muscle*. The detrusor is one of those muscles that our conscious brain does not really have a direct line on, and its actions are involuntary. Its job is to help the bladder fully empty its contents, so it adds a squeeze while we are urinating.

When the detrusor muscle gets overactive, it falls out of sync with how the bladder is functioning and it starts squeezing too soon and too often. There are a lot of different things that can affect how the detrusor is working. Sometimes this kind of overactivity is caused by drinking too much alcohol or caffeine. Dehydration can also cause the urine to concentrate in the bladder, which then becomes irritating to the detrusor. There are some medications that will also produce these same effects.

3. Combination Stress and Urge Incontinence

The third kind of incontinence is basically a combination of the two main types, stress and urge. This makes for a very touchy bladder situation in which the bladder and its environment are both fair game for causing us to leak. With this type of incontinence, we have to consider everything we drink and how well we are using our Inner Core. Many women try to control their leaking by reducing their fluid intake, but that is not a solution.

The good news is that, despite what most women think, it is possible to recover continence if you have lost control. There are a lot of helpful programs and information out there. Unfortunately, most women believe that this is just a part of life and they are too embarrassed to talk about it. The first step toward changing how your body works is to get information.

Pelvic Organ Prolapse

I consolidated incontinence with pelvic organ prolapse into this one chapter because there are a lot of interrelationships between these two issues, but they are not necessarily the same. They both involve the pelvic organs and how they function with the Pressure Mechanics of the Inner Core. However, it is possible to have incontinence and no signs of organ prolapse and vice versa. It is also possible to have both sets of problems.

Both incontinence and pelvic organ prolapse are associated with the two main events in a woman's body: pregnancy and menopause (with its concomitant aging). What is interesting is that there are women who experience both incontinence and prolapse but never had a baby. There are also women who have had babies and never develop either issue. So as you can see, there is more to these "facts of life" than what many women understand.

Pelvic organ prolapse is the protrusion or bulging of the pelvic organs into and/or through the walls of the vagina and the Pelvic Floor. The actual bulging of an organ into the vaginal walls has its own scientific name mentioned earlier: cele. There are a few different directions in which this can take place, each with its own name:

- Cystocele: when the bladder bulges or prolapses into the vagina.

- Rectocele: when the rectum bulges or prolapses into the vagina.

There are a few other variations of directions of prolapse that are useful to look into further if need be, and there are a lot of good organizations and websites that can provide that information.

There are four stages of prolapse:

- Stage 1 is a very mild case, in which the organs are still well supported by the Pelvic Floor.
- Stage 2 is indicated when the organs have fallen farther but are still contained in the vagina.
- Stage 3 is when the vaginal walls are no longer holding the organs and they have reached the opening of the vagina.
- Stage 4 is when the pelvic organs have fallen through the vaginal opening.

Once you understand exactly what a pelvic organ prolapse is and the different stages of it, it is easier to understand the relationships between incontinence and prolapse with pregnancy and menopause.

A Little More About the Floor

I have said this many times throughout this book, and I will say it again: The Inner Core muscles are amazing multitaskers. They have interesting arrangements of muscle fiber directions that hook into and rely on sheets of ligament and connective tissue. The Floor muscles are no exception in their own special complexity.

The Floor muscles have several special considerations in their construction that differ from the other muscles of the Inner Core. There are the gristly ligament connections, as well as the dense sheets of fascia that the Floor muscles rely on for support. These ligaments and fascia also support the urethra of the bladder, the vagina, and the rectum/anus. The muscles of the Floor generate tension that pulls on these ligaments and fascia in order to support the organs and maintain continence.

It is extremely important to understand this bit of Floor anatomy so that you can truly understand what aging and pregnancy have to do with incontinence and pelvic organ prolapse. Muscles are amazing because they have the ability to recover from most anything. If you can find it and contract it, it will change! Ligaments and fascia can restrengthen and restore; however, these structures do have a breaking point.

There are several things that can happen to tear or damage the ligaments and fascia of the Floor. There are direct traumas to the Floor itself that damage the ligaments and fascia. There is also the process of supporting a pregnancy and the actual birth of a baby. There is a multitude of other types of diseases and surgeries (outside the scope of this book) that affect how these things will work. If the ligaments and fascia have been too damaged, then the Floor may not be able to fully recover all of its dynamic capabilities.

The strength of the Floor is very dependent on its ligaments and fascia. Pelvic organ continence is dependent on the muscle ligament and fascia strength of the Floor. The ability of the organs to stay organized and not fall into the walls of the vagina depends on the muscle ligament and fascia strength of the Floor. However, the Floor does not stand alone. It needs the rest of the core to work well.

Core Pressure, Continence, and the Pelvic Organs

All women should have the opportunity to learn what's involved with how their Lady Business works. Change starts with how the muscles and pressure system work. When you know where these are and how they work, you can create change. This calls for a quick review of the Inner Core muscles and Pressure Mechanics.

All of the organs and circulatory systems are organized and supported in the abdominal area. These organs and systems are full of fluid, blood, and air and function very much like a water balloon. This water balloon relies on the muscle support of the Inner Core to hold its shape and function.

The Breather muscle is a kind of elastic plate that covers the top of the water balloon. It sandwiches the balloon with the elastic plate of the Floor muscle. This water balloon sandwich is then held together by the Encasement muscle. The tension of these three muscles supports

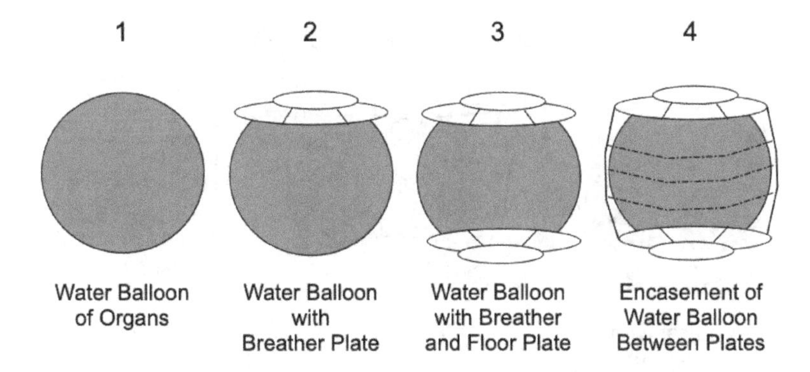

the water balloon, which is our internal pressure system. It's important to keep in mind that the bladder, uterus, and rectum live at the bottom of this pressure system.

Breath is driven by the Breather muscle, which is supported by the Encasement and the Floor. These three muscles control the pressure on and within the water balloon as well. When we inhale, the Breather muscle flattens and expands in order to draw air into the lungs. This expansion of the Breather muscle begins at the base of the ribs and follows through the abdomen all the way to the Floor. The Encasement muscle controls the abdominal expansion, and the Floor plate deepens to receive this breath expansion.

The flattening of the Diaphragm actually presses the entire organ system downward by as much as two centimeters. In order to prevent too much pressure on the organ systems, the Encasement and Floor muscles expand and deepen to control a descent of breath caused by the flattening of the Breather muscle.

Exhaling air is the reverse action. The Floor plate flattens and the Encasement draws back inward to move the organ system back to its starting position under the Diaphragm, which deepens back to its original position. All of these breath actions have various levels of tension depending on what we are up to. The key to health of the system is that the tension relationships among all three of these muscles remain balanced.

If the Breather muscle increases or changes its tension, then it puts more tension on the water balloon as well as on the Floor muscle. If

Pressure Mechanics of Breathing

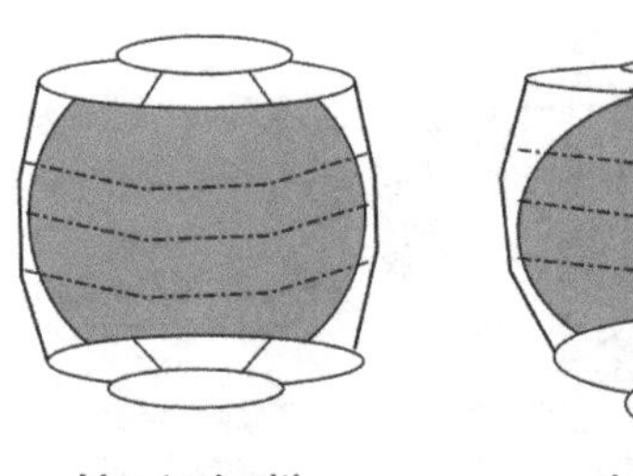

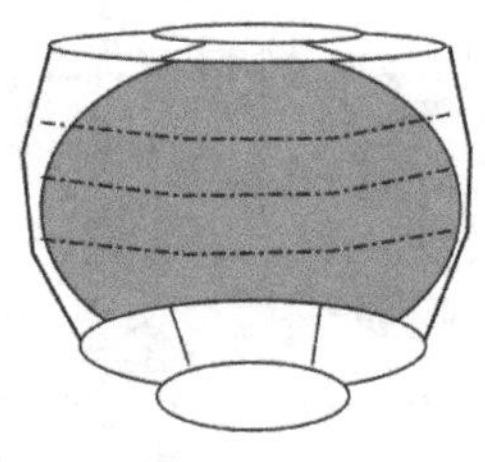

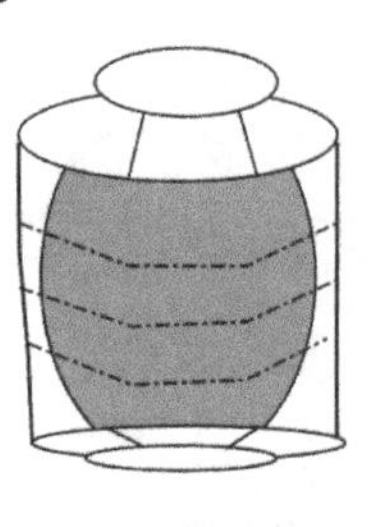

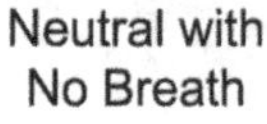

the Encasement muscle jumps up its tension and doesn't control the expansion, then there is more pressure on the Breather muscle as well as on the Floor. If the Floor is too tense, then it can't deepen and control the organ descent with breath, which causes the pelvic organs to become compressed.

Posture is also a big deal with pressure. I recently read the statistic that women with the slumped posture are 40 percent more likely to have a prolapse problem.

Does the slumped posture pictured here look familiar to you? This is the posture typically associated with older women, as it gets more pronounced with age. Despite what you have heard, this can be changed.

So, with all of this in mind, let's revisit what we know about stress incontinence. Continence relies on the entire pressure system working well and in harmony. The bladder needs a solid, well-coordinated Floor muscle to keep its urethra closed until we are ready to open it. The pelvic organs need to have a strong Pelvic Floor base. The pelvic organs do not need additional pressures from the Breather or other postural abdominal muscle pressures.

Bringing It All Together

Let's get back to some of the facts mentioned earlier. It is possible to have incontinence without ever having had a baby. It is possible to have a baby and never have incontinence. Same goes for organ prolapse.

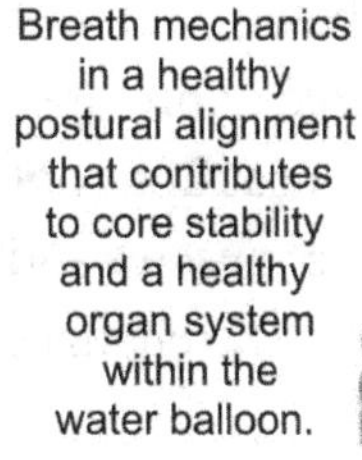

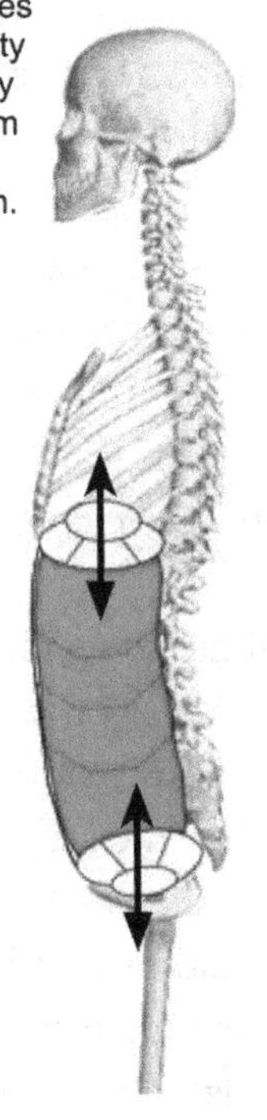

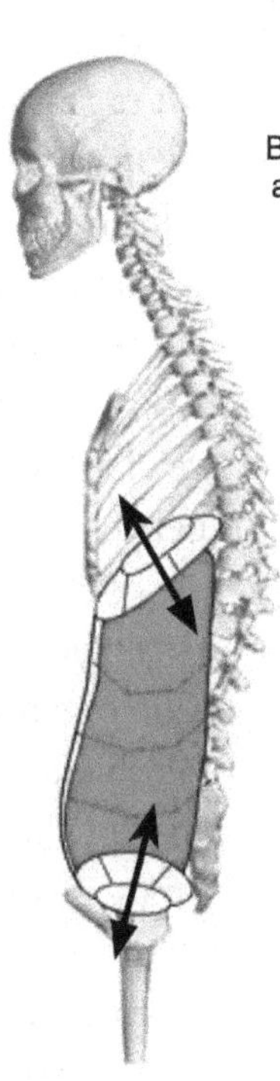

How is this possible, and what does it tell us? It's all about how the Inner Core muscles are working and how the pressure system is being supported and maintained.

Estrogen and other hormones affect how the strength and resilience of the ligaments and fascia work. Pregnancy has a special effect on this strength and resiliency because the woman's body needs to expand and flex for the growing baby. So there are going to be some effects on all of the Inner Core muscles, which is normal.

The key to recovering from having a baby is restoring all of the aspects that changed from carrying a baby, and that means more than just abdominal strength. Postural changes happen with baby bulk, along with the loss of muscle coordination of the Breather, Encasement, and Floor muscles. When these things are not restored, then continence is impacted, leaving women with this problem throughout their lives.

Pregnancy and childbirth can also leave a mark on the ligamentous and fascial strength and integrity of the Floor. Some degree of prolapse can occur that will remain with us throughout our lives. That does not mean we are doomed. It means we must optimize how the muscles and pressure system work. Optimizing can help avoid some of the changes that happen with menopause.

The main thing that menopause alone causes is a change in the elasticity and resiliency of the ligaments and fascia throughout the entire body. It is this change that naturally occurs in the ligaments and fascia associated with the Pelvic Floor muscles that can lead to age-related incontinence and/or pelvic organ prolapse. It is the change that sets us up for how we age.

This is why other risk factors can contribute to women having incontinence and/or pelvic organ prolapse regardless of whether or not they carried a baby. Problems with chronic constipation, for example, cause women to have to push and bear down excessively to have a bowel movement—that involves a high tension of the Diaphragm working to push out fecal matter. Smoking, asthma, and chronic obstructive pulmonary disease (COPD) also contribute to incontinence and organ prolapse. Again, these issues are related to the high tension of the Diaphragm.

In summary, the main message is that there is hope. It is so important to have an understanding of how your Inner Core is working before starting a core training exercise program. Everybody benefits from core exercise; however, it is crucial to understand where your body is at in its functioning. The Inner Core muscles must be managing the pressure system well before the body will benefit from a more strenuous, demanding core exercise program.

CHAPTER 9

Asthma and Chronic Obstructive Pulmonary Disease

There are a variety of diseases that cause problems with the ability to breathe, which also has an effect on the way that the Breather muscle works. Good breath is vital not only to get oxygen into the body, but also because it impacts all of the other important functions that the Breather muscle is in charge of, along with the Pressure Mechanics.

Asthma is a disease that affects how the lungs work. When you inhale air, it travels through a very elaborate network of *bronchial tubes*, or air channels, within the lungs. Asthma is a condition in which these airways become inflamed and swell up, which then limits the ability of air to get through. The main symptoms of asthma are difficulty breathing, coughing, wheezing, and tightness in the chest.

No one really understands why some people have asthma and others don't, but it is a manageable problem. First, you have to see a medical provider who will diagnose you, figure out what kinds of medications will help control the asthma attacks, and identify all the triggers for an attack.

Interestingly enough, although we don't really understand the underlying mechanisms of asthma, research has started to report that there is a link between asthma and hormones—specifically, estrogen and progesterone. Women who have asthma will notice a difference in how easily their symptoms are triggered depending on their menstruation cycle.

Chronic obstructive pulmonary disease, more commonly referred to as COPD, is a diagnosis for a group of diseases that all have one thing in common: difficulty breathing. There are two main diseases that share this diagnosis: chronic bronchitis and emphysema. Quite a few people develop these problems as they age, usually past their sixties. These folks often have a history of asthma, and some of them are/were smokers. Formerly, the majority of people with COPD were men (mostly because males smoked more than females did), but more recent studies are showing that the smoking habit has increased in women and, consequently, so have breathing problems.

The symptoms of COPD are just like those of asthma—a lot of coughing and wheezing. People with COPD struggle with shortness of breath and have a tough time taking deep breaths. This limit on how much air can get in the lungs starts to affect the kinds of activities you can do and to what extent. It can get so bad that just going up a few stairs can make you pant.

So how do asthma and COPD change the way the core works? Because both COPD and asthma are conditions that make it tougher to get air into the lungs, the Breather muscle has to work harder to maximize air intake. Any muscle that has to work harder than it is used to will get stiff.

Body Changes with COPD and Asthma

A lot of research has been done to figure out what types of treatment or intervention are most effective for respiratory diseases, and a lot of discoveries have been made along the way. The medical field has clearly identified which medications improve breath function, as well as which irritants to avoid. We also know more now about how the physical body changes in people who struggle for breath on a regular basis.

There are evidently three major compensations in the body associated with asthma and COPD, all of which are related to making it easier to take a breath. The Diaphragm, or the Breather muscle, has a much higher work demand on it, so there are changes in this muscle over time. This effort of muscle also causes people to tend to adapt their posture so they can get air into the lungs more easily. More muscles

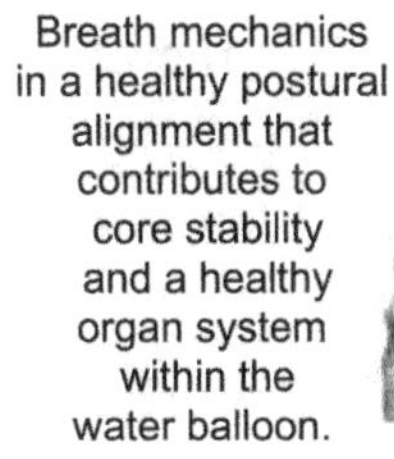

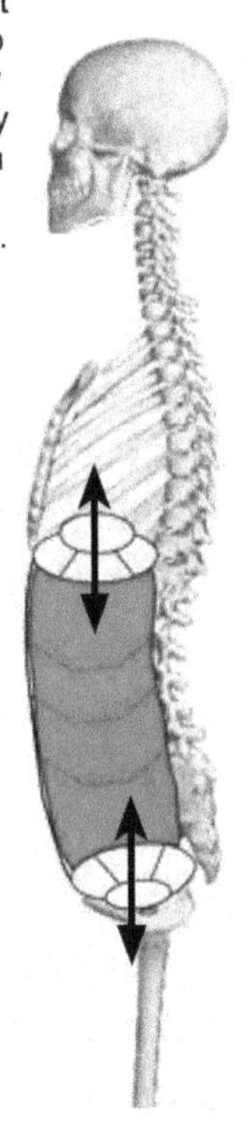

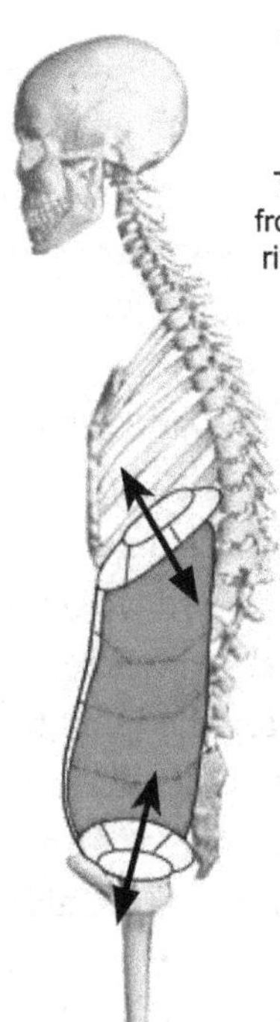

will get involved to help, which causes the shoulders, neck, and upper back to get stiffer.

The main consequence that drives all of the other changes is how the Breather muscle changes as a result of the struggle with breath. This muscle not only gets stiff, it tightens up and gets shorter and thicker. It loses elasticity over time, which not only changes its ability to do its job, but also its shape. It gets a little flatter. It also adds a lot more tension and compression to the water balloon organ system. Higher tension of a core muscle leads to more tension on the pressure system.

As mentioned, posture also changes significantly with the ongoing struggle to get air into the lungs. The body slumps down and the head juts forward, which almost seems counterintuitive to what you might expect. But this position gives the neck and shoulder girdle muscles the advantage of helping the Breather muscle get more air into the lungs.

Unfortunately, over time, these muscles change just like the Breather muscle does. The constant tension of working harder than they were engineered to do causes the muscles to shorten.

As the neck and shoulder girdle muscles adapt to these stressors of breath, the head and neck lose their ability to rotate, tip, and look up. The shoulder girdle muscles become strained in the back as the *pectoralis*—the chest muscles—become more and more stiff. This leads to the development of significant neck and shoulder pain over time.

All of these changes in posture of the head and neck cause the trunk to slump forward, which is actually very counterproductive for the Breather muscle. This muscle is also struggling, and this posture puts even more pressure on its ability to move through its full motion.

The more slumped we get, the harder it is to balance the body. This is a very big deal for women. The stiffer and more slumped you are, the harder it is for the body to stay upright, especially when you have to turn quickly to change directions or, heaven forbid, when you catch your foot on the edge of furniture. The stiffer you are, the more likely you will fall. This is so true across the spectrum of aging.

These changes in the adaptive shortening of the muscles, in combination with the posture changes, contribute to more stress on your Lady Business. Any condition that causes frequent coughing (as do asthma and COPD) is one of the top ten contributing factors to developing not only incontinence, but also pelvic organ prolapse. This fact can be hard to understand, especially if you don't have a coughing problem. But any woman who does knows how it feels to have that much pressure on their Lady Business, as well as the consequences of a nasty coughing attack.

What I just described is a common story of many aging women. First, they lose their posture, then their continence, then they trip and fall and break their hip. But this story can be interrupted—these changes can be addressed and improved. Women can greatly benefit from a good, comprehensive core training program. Studies have shown that even breathing ability can be improved. First, however, you must understand Pressure Mechanics and what must change first.

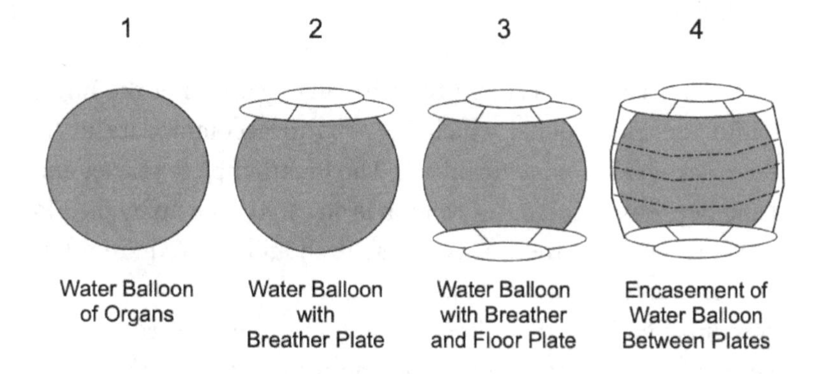

Core Consequences

A quick review of the Inner Core muscle system is called for yet again:

1. We can imagine all of the organs filled with air and fluid clustered around the main stem of blood vessels functioning a lot like a water balloon.
2. The Breather muscle covers the top of the water balloon and functions like an elastic plate.
3. The Floor muscle supports the bottom of the water balloon and also functions like an elastic plate.
4. The Encasement muscle wraps around the water balloon to support it between the sandwich of the two plates.

And now another look at breath within the Pressure Mechanics system:

Pressure Mechanics of Breathing

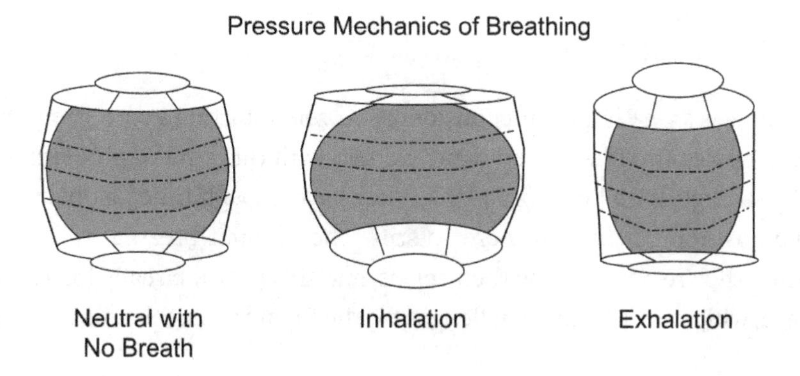

Inhalation involves the spreading and flattening of the Breather plate on the water balloon. As the breath increases its downward pressure, the water balloon is supported with an expansion of the Encasement into the Floor plate, which deepens to accommodate it. This process reverses with exhaling breath. The Breather plate relaxes and is lifted and deepens as the water balloon is elevated back up by the Floor plate with the help of the Encasement. It should not require a lot of work or tension for breath to happen.

Now imagine how the stiffening and shortening of the Breather muscle would put more pressure on the water balloon, the Encasement, and the Floor muscles. The constant push downward on the system puts a lot of pressure on the Floor. This is a huge consideration for the muscles and their connective tissues, as well as for the organs that live there. This is how asthma and COPD have become a risk factor for developing incontinence and Pelvic Floor prolapse in women.

You also have to remember that the Breather muscle is attached all the way around the base of the rib cage. When the Breather muscle gets stiff and flatter, it causes the cage to become more oriented in a slumped posture. This change in overall posture is yet another contributing factor to how one health condition can change core muscle function and Pressure Mechanics.

This is a great example of how these kinds of issues cause neck and back pain that is not that easy to stretch out. You cannot just stretch the body if it is being held there by a problem like asthma or COPD. You have to start with changing how the Breather muscle works in order to change how the rest of the body works.

Asthma and Core Training

Asthma is a very important consideration when starting a core strengthening program. I have seen many women with this kind of problem really struggle with holding a plank. They have a tough time just being in the position because they are so stiff. They cannot breathe well even when they're not exerting themselves, and this position really loads the cage, which causes more challenges for the Breather muscle to work. It's so important that these women start with stretching their bodies and working their Breather muscle before getting involved with planking.

I have a very good friend I've tried to help over the years with her chronic neck and shoulder pain. I've known her for quite a long time, about twenty years. She works as a physician assistant and loves to run, hike, and climb. She has bouts with asthma but is really good with her medical management. She started having a lot of neck and shoulder pain. Her shoulder started getting really stiff, so she reached out and started seeing me for physical therapy. The first thing I noticed about her was how stiff her upper back and rib cage were. This surprised me because she was so active. Usually, women that active are pretty flexible.

It took a long time to get her shoulder working better, and she eventually regained all of her motion. Unfortunately, her neck never fully recovered, and she continued to have bouts of severe pain that would come and go depending on how active she tried to be with her running. Considering how stiff her upper back was, it wasn't a surprise to me that she continued to have troubles with her neck. When you are that stiff in a slump, it puts an enormous amount of pressure and compression on the joint of the neck. She would come see me for treatment occasionally, and we tried everything. We put her through an intensive foam roller program, mobilization for her neck, shoulders, and back. After we worked, she could stand with better posture, but those gains never held.

She eventually let go of her running and hiking because they were just too painful, which was a huge disappointment to her. She resurfaced about two years ago because she was having so much pain that she could not comfortably walk or even turn her head. I noticed that her posture was also regressing and she was more slumped than before. She also mentioned that she was having a much harder time with her breathing capacity, getting short of breath just going up and down the stairs.

This time, we focused her rehabilitation on restoring her core because her posture and breath restriction were the sources of all her neck pain. Interestingly enough, she was very resistant to working with breath. It didn't make sense to her why this was a part of the core training. Her medical training was actually a barrier because these were new concepts for her. I had to pull out all of the research before she grudgingly agreed to try.

We started with getting her breath expansion back by focusing on increasing the length of her inhalations and exhalations. Lengthening the Breather muscle helps it become more flexible and dynamic. It also allows the cage as a whole to regain its flexibility. Now all of the stretching exercises for the cage could be more effective. Not only did my friend's posture improve along with her neck pain, but she also had much better breath capacity.

Special Considerations for Pelvic Organ Prolapse

The pelvic organs are at the bottom of the water balloon: the bladder, vagina, and rectum. When these organs are under a sustained amount of pressure, one or more of them can droop or prolapse onto each other and actually fall downward and out of the vagina. This is a very big deal for our Lady Business!

As we've talked about, there are surgeries that try to create restraints that hold these organs up, but their success rate over time is extremely poor. It's easier to understand why these procedures have limited long-term success and are largely unsuccessful when you consider that the biggest reasons why this happens to these organs are strongly related to the pressure of breath and poor coordination and control of the Inner Core. So women who develop a prolapse *and* have a medical condition like asthma or COPD must be handled with extra attention and care.

Restoring the Core in Individuals with Asthma or COPD

As I've said throughout, there is always hope with any of the conditions we've been discussing because we can always improve our core. We can improve not only the posture and flexibility of the body, but also the breath capacity of the Breather muscle. It's important to identify these issues early in the core training process because they direct the trainer, coach, or therapist as to where the program must begin.

The first thing is to restore normal inhalation. Women who have been compensating for so long have forgotten what that feels like. A normal inhalation begins with an expansion at the base of the cage, all 360 degrees of it. I compare it to opening an umbrella. A woman absolutely cannot use common cheating strategies like lifting the breastbone up to the chin or bearing down to force breath into the abdomen. Good, healthy breath is expansion, not just pushing into the belly.

It takes time to get the coordination right and restore the mobility at this stage. Mostly, I use manual techniques to help loosen up the neck and cage. A lot of stretching with good breath is required. You cannot progress into the strengthening process until you have restored the proper coordination to the Pressure Mechanics.

The next step I like to take with these women is to work with a resisted breath device, which basically resists air drawn in and blown out. Numerous studies have shown that exercise with this type of device makes a difference in how well the person with asthma and/or COPD can breathe. Once I feel that the breath and the pressure system are restored, I will then progress to the other exercises and activities for core training.

It is possible to make a difference in how the body can function with a good core training program. Women can improve their breath, their posture, and their balance—all key functions you want operating at their highest level in order to age successfully.

CHAPTER 10

Functional Gastrointestinal Disorders

Any medical condition that causes chronic, significant pain and bloating in the abdomen is unfortunately fair game for influencing the way our core muscles work. Pain is a powerful motivator, and muscles almost always have a response to it. Visceral pain is not different than any other source of pain, even though it is generated in the organs themselves. That is why these types of problems should be considered when you are working with a woman through the core training process.

Functional gastrointestinal disorders is a diagnosis category that describes changes in stomach/intestinal function that are not related to an actual structural or biochemical problem. Irritable bowel syndrome is the most common diagnosis of this type, and it basically means that there is an alteration in the bowel consistency and a lot of abdominal pain associated with it. It can result in either too much constipation, too much diarrhea, or a combination of both. People also always report experiencing a sense of bloating or distension with IBS. Research shows that women are typically more likely to have more trouble with the constipation type of IBS.

This category of medical conditions is another area in which problems seem to impact women more than men, which is another reason for devoting a chapter to it. Evidently, there's a multitude of issues that contribute to having and managing IBS. I found more than a few studies that discuss the relationship between estrogen and progesterone to flares of IBS. One study in particular notes that estrogen and progesterone actually cause an inhibition of smooth muscle, meaning these hormones will cause the smooth muscles of the intestines to slow down the contractions that move feces along (thus women's greater tendency to suffer from the constipation type of IBS).

I always rely on research when I educate people about how their bodies and their muscle systems work because evidence-based information is what should inform and drive our treatment decisions. What I want to explain about how the Inner Core and Pressure Mechanics change has been proven by research on people who have IBS. In my clinical practice working with ladies managing endometriosis and other issues that cause abdominal pain, I have seen some of these same changes.

Pain is a very powerful stimulus for changing how the muscles of the core function. We have a very primal response to brace against pain. This primal bracing includes changing the way we breathe, shortening the breath almost to a point of panting. Another reflex to pain is breath holding. There is something about visceral pain that invites that need to flex forward and hold, which almost feels like you are unloading that painful part.

The problem is that bracing and shortening of the breath cause a great deal of tension in the Diaphragm. The very mechanism that feels like it should help reduce the pain is actually causing more pressure and tension on what's causing the pain. Again, another counterintuitive response from our bodies, but a factual one nonetheless.

Core Consequences

Bear with me as we review once more the Inner Core's relationship to Pressure Mechanics because it's pertinent to this chapter's discussion of gastrointestinal problems:

1. We can imagine all of the organs filled with air and fluid clustered around the main stem of blood vessels functioning a lot like a water balloon.
2. The Breather muscle covers the top of the water balloon and functions like an elastic plate.

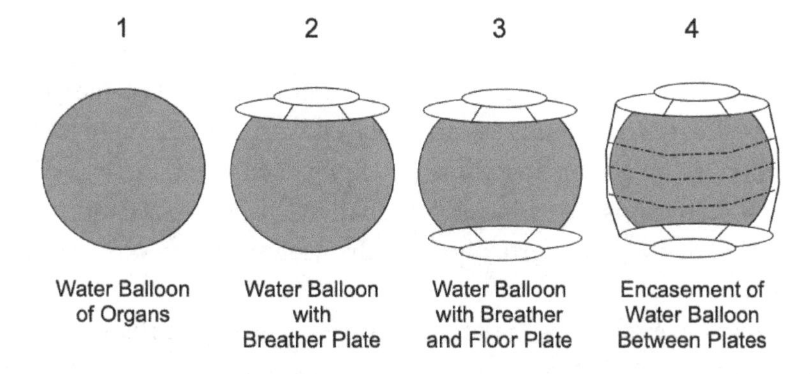

3. The Floor muscle supports the bottom of the water balloon and also functions like an elastic plate.
4. The Encasement muscle wraps around the water balloon to support it between the sandwich of the two plates.

Recall, also, this summary of how breath and Pressure Mechanics interact: Inhalation involves the spreading and flattening of the Breather plate on the water balloon. As the breath increases its downward pressure, the water balloon is supported with an expansion of the Encasement into the Floor plate, which deepens to accommodate it. This process reverses with exhaling breath. The Breather plate relaxes and is lifted and deepens as the water balloon is elevated back up by the Floor plate with the help of the Encasement. It should not require a lot of work or tension for breath to happen.

Pressure Mechanics of Breathing

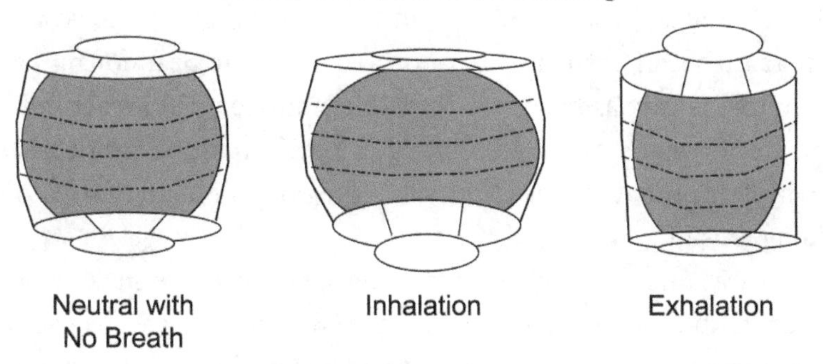

Abdominal Pain, Bloating, and the Core

Some really interesting research has been done in the last ten years or so on how the core muscles are involved with the whole process of digestion, as well as on how these muscles will change their activation patterns in response to eating. Although these changes in activation are somewhat subtle, they certainly make themselves known when we eat a big meal.

I think everybody can relate to that heavy feeling of fullness after eating a particularly big meal. This is always how I feel after the big turkey dinner on Thanksgiving, especially if I eat a lot of the foods that make me feel gassy later. The Inner Core muscles form the primary support for the organ system. So when a large quantity of food is delivered to the stomach and on down that intestinal line for digestion processing, that adds not only weight but also volume to the water balloon.

This additional volume, otherwise known as "the bloat," takes up space, and the Inner Core has to change its activation in order to accommodate that. Presumably, the normal response to bloating is a relatively minor relaxation of the Encasement, Oblique, and Breather muscles. This easing of tension levels helps accommodate the extra load and volume.

Interestingly enough, research has revealed that the activity response of the Inner Core muscles is quite different in people with IBS. In other words, when a bloating stimulus was induced in a group of people with IBS and a group of people with no functional gastrointestinal problems, a comparison of the reactions showed that the Inner Core behaved very differently in people with IBS. The Encasement and Obliques did relax a little, just as they did in the non-IBS group; however, the Diaphragm became much more tense and started to bear down.

Opinions vary as to why the Breather muscle would react in a way opposite to what's expected. One of the main reasons for this has to do with the primal response to pain—the body's bracing for pain and holding tension.

Lisa was referred to me for physical therapy because she was having a lot of trouble with pain in her low back and pelvis, as well as pain with sex. She was about thirty-two when I met her and had not developed any problems with continence. She also wanted to have a baby but was very concerned about how her back and pelvis would be affected by pregnancy.

Lisa's issues with back and pelvic pain were very obviously related to her posture and very poor core muscle function. She was extremely slumped. In fact, she was so slumped that, from the side, she looked like the letter *C*. A posture this extreme puts a lot of stress and strain on the connective tissue that holds the spine and pelvis together, as well as the muscles of the back.

Some of the other chapters have talked about how this type of posture affects the internal pressure system. All of that weight of the cage dropped forward like that puts a lot of load onto that pressure system, which increases that amount of pressure within it, which then puts a lot of pressure compression onto the pelvis and its Floor muscle. This causes the Floor muscles to get overused, which in turn causes pelvic pain and pain during sex.

The really interesting piece of Lisa's story was what was causing her to become so restricted in that posture. She had pain in her stomach throughout most of her life. There was not an obvious structural reason for why she had this pain, so she relied on over-the-counter medications to help her when she ate for the last twenty years or so of her life.

That chronic pain had caused a lot of bracing. Not only did she lose the elasticity and movement of her Breather muscle, but she also developed what we call *adaptive shortening* of the Outer Core muscles—when the Six-Pack and Oblique muscles become extremely tight, to the point where they actually shorten. So Lisa's problem with her back pain actually was an indirect result of her stomach pain. She had tried many different therapies to get relief from her back pain, but nothing ever seemed to change it. She even tried core exercise but fortunately discontinued it when she started hurting more.

The reason why all of the other therapies were unable to change Lisa's pain and posture was because treatment wasn't directed to where her back problem began. The changes in the core muscles because of her chronic stomach pain had to be addressed before anything else could be changed. We started with restoring the flexibility and coordination of her Breather muscle. Some patients have a tough time understanding how breath exercises can actually help with back and pelvic pain, but Lisa was willing to try anything by the time I started seeing her. Once her Breather muscle function started to improve, she was able to regain some control over her posture.

She had to do quite a bit of stretching of all of the core muscles, and she had to learn how to control her tendency to hold her breath. When people get in the habit of breath holding during motion or with exertions, they don't even realize that they are doing it. Lisa was very motivated to change her pain, so she was very consistent with her exercise and her habit modification.

Lisa did great with therapy and with resolving her pain. As we were able to get her stretched out, we started introducing other core exercises to her routine. She was able to change her posture, fully resolve her back pain, and eliminate pain with sex.

There Is Hope

Problems with digestion, bloating, and gas are extremely frustrating, so a lot of people try every diet that offers a whisper of hope to alleviate these symptoms. Many studies I've read started looking at how the Inner Core muscles respond to gut and stomach pain, and consideration is being given to the possibility that this reaction of tension and bearing down of the Breather muscle might be part of the problem for IBS sufferers in particular.

Lisa's stomach pain did not really change as her core function and breathing improved, although all of her other symptoms responded well. It could be because her stomach problem was not really an IBS issue, even though she struggled with the same pain and bloating associated with IBS. Two of the studies I reviewed about IBS applied the same kind of training I did, aiming to restore the Breather muscle's flexibility and function in these patients. The results demonstrated a reported change in pain levels as well as less bloat.

Any type of functional gastrointestinal disorder needs to be identified in any woman who is starting a core exercise training program. Lisa's story aptly reflects that this kind of problem does not respond well to just planking and crunching. Her situation required some stretching and coordinating of the Inner Core, which is the case most of the time for many women.

CHAPTER 11

Back Pain

Back pain is one of the many motivators that drive people to get involved with core training. After all, it makes sense that having a strong core will protect your back. That is true. It will protect your back. However, like everything else with the body, there is more to that story.

In chapter 5, we talked a lot about the consequences of back pain when you start a core training exercise program that is focused on just planking and crunching without first restoring core muscle function. There are a lot of different health issues that can cause changes in how the Inner Core and Outer Core muscles are working. Having a spinal injury, for example, causes significant changes in how the core muscles work.

There are also a lot of reasons why people experience back pain. But no matter the cause, it can be a debilitating situation because when your back hurts, it's hard to even get out of bed and stand up. Pain can come from problems with disc herniation, osteoarthritis, bone spurs, compression fractures, and even the muscles and connective tissue. All of these types of problems require exercise, but it's just like with everything else: It has to be the right exercise at the right time for the right problem.

I see problems like this every day in the clinic. The reason I focus my practice on chronic spinal and pelvic problems is because every patient is unique in what's going on with them. I find it so interesting to figure out how the muscles are responding to the pain situation. You must know what muscle is tensing up to protect the spine problem and what muscle is compensating for it. Every patient is like a puzzle to solve. They can have the same diagnosis, but no body reacts to pain the same way.

Many women suffering with back pain go to their doctor and are advised to take up yoga or Pilates. Sometimes that works out, but a high percentage of these ladies end up with more problems than they started with. Most of the time, the original pain levels go up. Sometimes they start having more trouble somewhere else in their body. Sometimes they develop more trouble with continence.

The experience of back pain can cause significant changes in how the core muscles function. Activation patterns of several core muscles are altered, and when the patient is stuck in pain for a few months, then the muscle memory of the involved core muscle is altered.

Back Facts

The best way to explain back pain and how it affects core muscles is to start with explaining the spine and how it works. The spine is a stack of bones. At the top of this stack of bones is the head, which itself sits on the top of the seven bones known as the *cervical bones*, or neck bones. Next, there are twelve *thoracic bones* that have the ribs attached to them. The bottom five bones form the *lumbar region*. All of these bones are stacked on top of the *sacrum*, the triangular-shaped bone in the center of the pelvic ring.

All of these bones make up the house for our nervous system, which is the most important structure of the entire body. It's important because it is in charge of everything in our lives. In fact, it's in charge of living. The brain lives in the skull, and it has a spinal cord that comes off the base. This spinal cord travels down through the central hole in each bone of the spine. The entire bony spinal column encases the cord. In between each bone, a pair of nerves comes off either side of the cord to exit the spine through the side holes.

In between each bone is a disc that's like a jelly donut. The jelly center is mostly comprised of a gel-like water. The cake part of the donut holds this gel center and is made of a very thick gristle that attaches all around the periphery of the body of the bone. That disc is firmly attached in between each bone. It doesn't "slip out" like some people think.

Behind the disc is the main central hole for the spinal cord, as well as side holes from which the nerves exit. Behind those holes is where you will find the joints of the spine. These joints are different than other joints of the body. They are basically bony knobs that slide open and shut, one on top of the other. There are two facet joints at each level that slide and glide with the bone above and the bone below.

All these bones are held together in a big stocking of ligament, which, you will recall, is another form of gristle. It's thick and dense and binds the bones together, but it also has a little flex to it so that the spine can bend and twist.

As the house for the entire nervous system, the spine has a lot of demands put on it. One of its responsibilities is to carry the brain and its parts around vertically. The spine house is always under the load of gravity until it lies down in bed. The spine also has to bend and twist in all directions. It is an amazing feat of engineering because it is built to do a lot of different things.

Spinal motion is considered *segmental*—that means each bone contributes to motion. Each bone of the spine tips forward and backward. They also have to tip sideways and rotate. They're able to do this because of the gel donut disc that's in between each bone.

When we bend forward, one bone rocks forward on top of the other one. The body of the bone compresses the front wall of the donut and stretches the back wall. The hole where the nerve comes out gets bigger, and both of the joints slide open. When we bend backward, the opposite happens. The bone rocks backward, compressing the back wall of the disc and stretching the front wall. The hole where the nerve comes out gets smaller, and both of the joints slide shut. When you side bend, one side compresses and the other side opens. Rotating compresses one joint and gaps the other.

All of this segmental action is happening at every bone when you bend over to reach the floor or twist around to reach behind you. That's a lot of moving parts! All those moving parts have to be controlled. It gets particularly challenging to control the bones when bending happens simultaneously with twisting and reaching. So what is actually controlling these moving bones? What is supporting and holding these bones together besides just the ligaments?

It's All About the Core

Core muscles. All of this holding and controlling of the bones happens because of the core muscles. Each one of these muscles has a job to do, and all of the other muscles rely on it. In other words, when one muscle isn't participating like it should, then the other muscles have to compensate for that. If one muscle is too tight and tense, then the other muscles become strained and have to make up for it.

A favorite therapist saying in the clinic is the old familiar "What came first, the chicken or the egg?" Posing this question represents the challenge of figuring out which muscle triggered what reaction when we're working to restore core muscle function. Did the Encasement muscle become weak and the Six-Pack muscle compensate for this and become extremely tense and painful? Did the Back Strap get strained and tight because all the abdominal muscles were not activating with lifting a lot of weight repeatedly?

There is a tension relationship among all these muscles. Recall the guy wire analogy I presented in chapter 2—how you see baby trees being supported out along highways or on lawns. Each guy wire has a certain amount of tightness that is countered by the opposite guy wire. The tension levels of the guy wires have equal and opposite pulling tension on the baby tree. If one guy wire is pulling more than any other, then the baby tree would list to the side of the strongest-pulling guy wire.

This is also true in the core, although the relationship is much more dynamic. If you cut the Six-Pack guy wire, then the Back Strap would be unopposed and the body would perpetually extend backward. If you cut the Back Strap, then the Six-Pack would be unopposed and the body would bend over.

Again, the core muscle system is far more dynamic than a simple guy wire system; however, the tension relationship is like that. The core is more dynamic because it has to do more than just hold the bones upright like a baby tree. The core needs to hold the bones, move the bones in all the different directions, hold and support the organs and their pressures, breathe, and manage continence.

That's a Big Job

That's a lot of action to consider controlling. And what's in charge of all that? The brain and nervous system. How can the brain coordinate all those actions? When you consider that every day, we humans are bending, lifting, and twisting while standing or walking and breathing and holding our pee at the same time, that's just too much to think about.

All of that can happen because of the concept of muscle memory. Every muscle of the body has a nerve attached that fires the muscle to make it contract. If there is no nerve connected, then there is no muscle contraction. There is a nerve that contracts the muscle that comes down from the brain and hooks into the muscle. There is also a nerve that comes from the muscle and goes up into the brain to tell the brain what the muscle is actually doing.

Both of these nerves to each muscle have a specific section in the brain where they connect. As you may recall from our discussion in chapter 4, these sections are mapped. The brain has a map—the motor map—for every nerve that goes to every muscle to make it contract. There is another map—the sensory map—for every nerve that tells the brain about what every single muscle is doing.

These maps interact with other parts of the brain that are involved with memory. This is how muscle memories become established. From the time that we are little babies, muscle memories are encoded in the brain. This is how we just raise our arms to shampoo our hair in the shower and unload the dishwasher without having to even think about these actions. Our brain has already encoded and learned the sequencing of muscle action and reaction.

Muscle memory includes the different movements of the different muscles that are involved with whatever action you want to take. This equates to the amount of tension of the muscle, along with the precise timing of when the muscle is supposed to kick on and off in conjunction with other muscles kicking on into contraction.

The process of developing a muscle memory takes time and practice. It's kind of like when you first learn to ski. The brain has no memory of how to work the muscles when you are on a pair of skis, so it has to learn. When we first try something new, we feel extremely awkward and clumsy. We don't know how much tension is required to hold the skis straight or pivot for the turns. The balance feels all wrong and we fall over easily.

After a certain amount of practice, though, the brain starts to learn what kind of tension each muscle needs and how to sequence the muscles for different actions. This kind of learning is the development of muscle memory. The more memories the brain stores, the less concentration is required. This is how we go from a rigid death grip on the ski poles, fearing for life and limb, to smooth, fluid moves, curving side to side down the trail while laughing with friends. Practice and muscle memory.

Problems with the Spinal House

As I've made clear, I get a lot of fulfillment from working with patients with back and pelvic pain because each unique case affords me the opportunity to find the precise source of the pain and then devise a plan to resolve it. When you are examining a patient with back pain, you are evaluating the house of the nervous system and brain. The house has sustained some kind of damage, and the brain is extremely protective of its house. The brain responds to damage by ramping up tension of the muscles in order to protect itself. Your job as a therapist is to determine what muscles are protecting the house and why. Then you must figure out what muscles are compensating for the protection. There are several different types of house damage.

Strains and sprains. There is a multitude of scenarios in which a strain or a sprain can happen to the spine. A sprain occurs when the ligament stocking of the spine is damaged. A strain occurs when the muscle is damaged. These injuries are usually related to an actual trauma. This could be anything from lifting a heavy weight when you are too tired to a slip and a fall to a car accident. It's just like a strain or sprain anywhere else in the body. These structures become inflamed and painful, and it takes a while for that to settle down. Once the inflammation is better, then the muscle and ligament need help to regain their strength.

Disc herniation. When a disc herniates, the outer gristly section of the disc breaks down and the gel center protrudes. This problem is referred to in varying ways—a "bulging disc," a "disc protrusion," or a "ruptured disc"—depending on the severity of the damage. The outer gristle can break down anywhere along its circumference. Most of the time, it happens along the back side because that wall is most commonly under load with bending. When the disc is damaged, it becomes inflamed and swells up. The swelling and bulging occupy space in the actual house. This swelling and bulging threaten the spinal cord and nerves. The brain doesn't like it when its cord or nerves get pinched or squeezed, so it drives the tension levels of the muscle up to protect itself.

Osteoarthritis. Arthritis of the spine involves the actual thinning of the cartilage that lines the joints, as well as thinning of the discs. This condition is usually labeled "degenerative joint disease" or "degenerative disc disease." It is a natural process of aging that happens to everybody. Arthritis doesn't always cause pain, although it quite often gets the blame for it. Arthritis can become a source of pain when the thinning of the joints or discs starts to threaten the cord or nerves. It's all about the space in the house. If the thinning causes too much settling of the house, then the holes where the nerves come out can get too small.

Spinal stenosis. The word "stenosis" literally means a narrowing of a passage. In this instance, it's describing the narrowing of the holes of the spine. There is a *central stenosis*, which is the narrowing of the central hole in which the spinal cord lives. *Foraminal stenosis* is the narrowing of the holes where the nerves come out of the house. These holes usually become narrowed by the buildup of bone spurs. Bone spurs are formed as the arthritic thinning of the cartilage and disc changes. When there is a history of damage to the spine, these bone spurs are usually bigger. How a spur forms and how big it gets determine how much of a threat the spur is to the cord and nerves.

Muscle Memory and Pain

All of the different types of spine problems are actually about the space in the house. When the house gets too crowded, then the brain gets worried. The crowding can be mostly inflammation, which involves swelling. The brain must protect its parts by tension guarding and bracing with a few chosen core muscles, depending on where the swelling is. If it's the house that gets crowded by arthritic changes and spurring, then the tension guarding and bracing turn up.

The main reasons the brain changes how the muscles of the core are working involve pain, inflammation, and the threat of crowding the house. All of the muscles' memories are stored in the brain. This is where those patterns of how the muscles work are altered. The brain is very protective of its nervous system parts. The brain cord and nerves are very unforgiving of being compressed or squeezed in any way. As a result, there are a lot of reactions and reflexes that are protective.

This is why I have a job! All of this protective guarding and muscle memory change makes it very difficult to recover from a significant injury to the spine. Some of these changes follow people throughout their lives. Their pain problems keep flaring up and tend to get worse over time.

It is truly a vicious cycle. Pain and inflammation cause the muscles to tense up and guard to protect. The high tension of the muscles puts more pressure on the spine and its discs and cartilage. This extra pressure feeds into the pain and inflammation, which causes more high-tension protective guarding. Around and around it goes, and it can become very difficult to break the cycle.

Treatment of such problems can begin to break the cycle. Finding a way into reducing the pain and relieving the tension guarding cycle is a challenge that can be addressed in multiple ways. This is where things like massage, electrical stimulation, acupuncture, and traction are all helpful in reducing guarding and muscle spasm—which in turn decreases the pain.

The next step that should happen is investigating what muscle memories have been disrupted. Change in muscle memory can go in two directions. You can have *inhibition*, which is a weakness of the muscle.

The muscle was turned off and so the memory dropped down. Then there's *alteration* of the muscle memory, which involves overactivation. The muscle was held in a state of high tension for so long that this tension became its new memory.

There are other changes of the core muscles in response to pain. Breath holding is a big deal as well. Holding your breath in response to pain is very common. It's also a great way to compensate for the weakness of the core. Unfortunately, it changes how the pressure system is loaded and adds more loading.

There are also changes in posture in response to pain. Sometimes the pain and swelling make it impossible to stand completely straight. This forces the muscles to change how they work. Even when the swelling goes away, the new habit of being bent forward remains in the muscles.

The Core Must Be Restored for Back Pain Relief

Back pain can be very challenging to resolve. The spine is a very complicated system with a lot of built-in strategies for compensation, which is great until you run out of space. The toughest thing about treating these kinds of conditions is figuring out what isn't doing its part.

I have seen a lot of spines that have significant disc problems and bone spurring but can still work well without pain. Just because the disc changes or there is a lot of narrowing doesn't mean that it can't still work. It's all about muscle control. If the core muscles are all doing their jobs and working in harmony, then the house will be okay.

There are steps to this process. Once the initial cycle of pain and spasm is settled down, then the inhibited weak muscle needs to be brought on line and the high-tension guarded muscles must be stretched. Breath must work well. All of this must come together for the posture to resume its natural alignment.

The type of generic program you might find in a standard yoga or Pilates class is sometimes not helpful, and there are reasons for this. If the problem is minor and you just need a little strength training or stretching, a generic program can be helpful. Unfortunately, this isn't the right place to start for many people, though it is a great option for continuing to maintain your fitness after your core has been restored.

CHAPTER 12

Osteoporosis

One of the more common things I have heard women worry about is getting a "hump" in their back as they get older. This hump, also known as a "hunchback" or "dowager's hump," is synonymous with looking like an old lady. Women ask me all the time what exercises will get rid of that hump. This chapter clarifies just what that formation is all about and how it relates to osteoporosis.

Let's start with *osteoporosis* itself, defined as "a systemic skeletal disease characterized by low bone mass and micro-architectural deterioration of bone tissue with a consequent increase in bone fragility and susceptibility to fracture." What that means is that the structure of the bones changes and weakens as women get older, especially after menopause.

Bones are not as hard and solid as they seem. They are made up of a network of dense collagen and other types of special proteins. This collagen and protein make up a matrix of sorts that hosts different minerals. The minerals are what make the bone strong and able to carry a lot of weight, and the collagen is what gives the bone some flex and shock absorption.

Bones don't stop growing when we stop growing. They don't get longer or wider; however, they are always responding to the stress placed on them. They are constantly remodeling and repairing themselves throughout the entire life cycle. They are able to do this with certain types of cells called *osteoblasts* and *osteoclasts*. Osteoblasts build the bone up and osteoclasts melt it down. Both are important for the repair process that is constant throughout life.

Estrogen is a very important hormone to the health and strength of the bones. Estrogen, along with a few other hormones, influences the way osteoblasts and osteoclasts work. When the body slows down the production of estrogen, this changes how the osteoblasts and osteoclasts function, which results in bone that becomes brittle and fractures more easily. A little trip and fall could cause a bone with osteoporosis to break.

There are several reasons why a woman might get osteoporosis. The most well-known reason is simply getting older, which includes the drop in estrogen levels. There are also dietary reasons—not getting enough calcium or other minerals in your diet. There are some health conditions that require women to take glucosteriods for long periods of time. Osteoporosis is a side effect of that kind of medication.

What's Up with the Hump?

So back to the hump! The hump we associate with getting older develops long before we might get osteoporosis. It's all about the posture. Posture is a habit, and it's tough to change bad habits. I find that when most people try to change their posture, they start in the wrong place. We have all heard, "Pull your shoulders back and straighten up!" Believe it or not, that's not the best place to start (which we'll discuss later in the chapter).

Not all women develop a hump as they age. Some women hold their posture well throughout their life—that is, if they're using their Inner Core well and managing to avoid traumas. Not all women who get osteoporosis develop a hump—that is, if they're able to optimize the care of their bone health and avoid falls and fractures.

The hump is basically an indication of loss of postural control of the head, spine, cage, and pelvis. Good posture isn't just about always holding a straight back. It's about having the ability to more or less hold your pelvis over your legs and stack a neutral cage over the pelvis. The head and shoulders literally organize themselves over that cage and pelvis.

It's also okay to drop down into a slump or move into a big arch. The main point is that you should be able to retain the ability to get into the alignment just described and sit comfortably with it for a sustained period of time. To stand up and walk with this alignment without adding more tension or stress to hold it. To bend over to pick up your cat and then be able to carry your cat out the door holding that alignment, assuming your cat weighs ten to fifteen pounds—if we're talking your fifty-pound dog, well, that will require some accommodation of posture on your part.

There are two distinct changes in proper alignment that are considered *not* optimal posture. One is a tipping of the pelvis forward and the cage up with a big arch in the back (you will notice that the shoulders have no choice but to drop back as a double chin appears). The other is more of what we associate with a hump, when the pelvis tucks under, the cage slumps forward, and the spine curves in. The shoulders have no choice but to round forward and the head juts out.

These postures have been illustrated earlier in the book, when we talked about how they not only rob us of full breath and core power, but also contribute to developing problems with the muscles and the organs within the pressure system. The slumped posture is what people think of as a hump. That's all it is—a hump related to the slump—a muscle memory problem of the core that creates more stress on the bones and muscles and more pressure in our organ system.

If you go through your forties and fifties with these changes in your posture and in your muscle memory, that's what sets you up for a much higher potential for complications from osteoporosis. There's no new or different hump that pops up because you have osteoporosis. It's the same one you already had that will get potentially much worse.

Osteoporosis and the Hump

To bring this all together so that it makes sense, we need to talk a little bit about biomechanics and how the bones of the spine and cage carry our weight. In other words, we need to talk about gravity. Gravity is a blessing and a curse. It's a blessing because science tells us that we need to load our bones to stimulate our osteoblasts to make more bone collagen. It's a curse because when we let our posture give way to the slump hump, then gravity loads our bones differently—and not in a good way.

Our spine and cage form a beautifully engineered stack of bones. This stack of bones houses our nervous system. It holds the trunk and head of the body upright against gravity, and it moves in 360 degrees of direction. We would not be able to bend and twist very well if any of these bones were shaped differently.

There is a curve to the spine, and it's there for a good reason. The rib cage is a heavy set of bones. It is much easier and more efficient to carry that heavy cage over the pelvis. If the spine were stick straight, then we would tip forward. Not only that, we wouldn't be able to reach up very well with our arms because our shoulders would be way out in front of our head.

The bones of the upper back are called the *thoracic vertebrae*. The front part of the vertebrae is called the *vertebral body*. This is where the majority of the weight of the body loads through the bone when we are upright. The thoracic upper-back bones normally carry this body weight a little more to the front of the vertebral body. When we slump, there is even more body weight in the front of the bone.

When we get in bad posture habits and slump all the time, all of our connective tissues and muscles adapt to that. The muscles of the front of the body shorten and lose their ability to flex; the muscles of the back of the body have to work much harder to control the stack of bones. Like I said, the cage is heavy, and it's a lot of work to hold it when it droops down.

Many people believe that the slump hump cannot be changed once it's there, but that's not true—to a certain point, at least. For those people who develop osteoporosis, there *is* an actual point of no return. All of that loading of the front of the thoracic vertebral body becomes a real problem when we get osteoporosis. Remember how estrogen drops and the bone matrix gets weakened and loses its mineralization? The front of the thoracic vertebral body literally starts to compress into a wedge shape. This is also how compression fractures occur. The front part of the vertebral bone collapses, and there is no getting that bone back to its original form.

There is a distinct difference in the appearance of a hump related to slumped posture versus an osteoporosis-related hump that has become a permanent fixture because of a compression wedge fracture. In the latter, the curvature of the hump becomes more rounded, and it's very difficult to straighten or reach up. Unfortunately, this kind of hump can lead to developing more compression fractures. The greater the curvature, the more pressure focuses on the front of the thoracic vertebral body. The more pressure of this nature, the more likely the bone will fracture.

These ladies are really stiff in their bodies. This kind of stiffness in the spine makes it easier to fall. The stiffer you are, the more likely you will fall. A stiff, forward-bent spine makes it more difficult to move all the way down to the feet. These women tend to drag their feet more. They also sway more side to side. It becomes easier to catch your foot on a rug or furniture. Once you start to tip, there is no wiggle room in which to catch yourself. Balance is all about having wiggle room. When we lean too far out over our small center of gravity, we should be able to wiggle or tip the head and upper back over to shift our body weight back over the center of gravity.

If You Fracture, There Is Still Hope!

If you develop osteoporosis and sustain a compression fracture of your thoracic spine, there is still hope that you will not end up permanently bent over. There is a cascade of events following a fracture that leads to that end, and it can be prevented. However, it does require an investment of time, energy, and exercise.

The first thing that happens after a fracture occurs is that you have to take it easy and let the fracture heal. Sometimes this involves wearing a big clamshell of a brace that keeps the body from bending and putting pressure on the bone structure. Taking it easy is tough on the body because when we aren't using our bodies, we get weak. Our muscles lose strength, as does the connective tissue and gristle that holds the bones together. We also lose our cardiovascular fitness and get winded more easily.

The second thing that happens after a fracture is that you hurt, and this makes you scared. Feeling so fragile gets in the way of getting moving again. There is also the desire to brace yourself with your muscles and hold your breath, both of which contribute to yet more stiffness.

After a fracture, it is extremely important to consult a skilled physical therapist or trainer who will guide you back to good coordination, flexibility, and fitness. A big part of successfully aging with osteoporosis is making your fitness program a regular element in your daily self-care and lifestyle. It's kind of like brushing your teeth—you just devote a certain part of your day to brushing your teeth because you know it's a vital part of maintaining your overall health.

I always tell my patients that although exercise does require some degree of thought in terms of technique, pacing, and so forth, it's not rocket science. The hardest thing about exercise and fitness activities is making time for them. At what time of day are you most likely to make it happen on a consistent basis? Some ladies prefer morning and some prefer evening. You need to find a space for it in your life and then hold that space.

Important Considerations

This section of this chapter is extremely important for all women who know they have osteoporosis, for women over fifty who might have osteoporosis but aren't sure, and for any trainers, therapists, Pilates/yoga instructors, or fitness techs who are working with these women. There are certain things to keep in mind because, after all, exercise and fitness are supposed to benefit health, not contribute to more problems. There is no specific type of pain or soreness that tells you that you might have osteoporosis.

It's tricky because our current science and diagnostic tools do not necessarily tell us who will get a compression fracture and who won't. A DEXA scan can definitively indicate osteoporosis, but sometimes other things can cause fractures—risk factors that increase the likelihood of having this kind of problem. These risk factors include:

- Being a female over the age of 50
- Being a very thin female of low body weight
- Having gone through menopause
- A family history of developing osteoporosis
- A history of rheumatoid arthritis
- Any condition that requires ongoing steroid medication
- Any history of breast/ovarian cancer treated with tamoxifen or another medication that inhibits estrogen production

So, if you are a therapist, trainer, Pilates/yoga instructor, or fitness tech who has a lady walking into your clinic, gym, or studio, these are the things you'll want to know about her—the risk factors that apply to her. Once you have this knowledge, you can not only incorporate certain exercises into your program to address them, but you can avoid certain activities that could cause trouble for them.

Fitness fanatic Amber was seventy-two, with rheumatoid arthritis. I had seen her in the past for various problems with back pain. She really enjoyed exercise and was always involved with some kind of fitness program. Amber also had a history of breast cancer and had been taking tamoxifen for ten years. She came to see me because she started to develop pelvic pain after exercising with her trainer.

I immediately mentally logged all of Amber's risk factors for osteoporosis: the steroids she took to treat her arthritis, the estrogen-depleting medication she took to treat her cancer, and her extreme thinness. When she told me about the different things she was doing with her trainer, I politely asked her to discontinue this relationship and work with someone else. Most of the elements of her program were good exercises; however, she was doing a lot of breath holding during her core exercises and she was squat lifting and dead lifting up to seventy pounds. Although she was able to do these exercises fairly well and did not have any pain (until she did), it's just not a good idea to load up a little lady this much. It was kind of asking for trouble.

It turned out that most of Amber's pain was actually related to the higher pressure of lifting that amount of weight and to the breath holding during it, which was causing additional pressure on her reproductive organs and bladder. So there were elements of visceral pain, as well as a lot of pressure on the pelvic ligaments, which was also painful. She did not sustain a compression fracture—fortunately, but also a little bit surprisingly. I personally felt grateful that she'd developed the kinds of pains that are easier to fix. It was these pains that brought her back to my office so I could help her and then redirect her to a better and safer trainer.

It is really important to be cautious with these ladies and their exercises. High levels of bracing and breath holding with lifting and reaching can cause increased co-contraction of core muscles, which increases pressure on the vertebral bones. It is also important to moderate the amount of weight these women are lifting in a forward flexion motion. That direction of lifting can cause more compression on the front part of the thoracic vertebral body.

These ladies also really need to maintain their flexibility and breath. Breath exercise helps keep the ribs of the cage moving, and it's a core exercise. There are a ton of reasons I've discussed throughout this book as to why we need to keep our Diaphragm flexing through its full excursion. There is a lot of power that comes from breath with motion. Flexibility and breath are synonymous with balance.

PART THREE

RESTORE YOUR INNER CORE

CHAPTER 13

Evaluate Your Core

Hopefully by this point in the book, you have a good understanding of how the core muscles work, of the Pressure Mechanics of our organ system, and of the consequences of an out-of-control core. In order to move forward with learning how to assess your own Inner Core, ask yourself these questions:

1. What does the core have to do with the Floor?
2. Why do we care about how we breathe?
3. What is the internal pressure system?
4. Which muscles are in charge of the pressure system?
5. What is more important: strength or coordination?
6. How does the pressure system affect core function?

The Pelvic Floor muscles literally form the floor of the core. In other words, they're the base plate for the entire core system. What happens in the core directly affects how the Floor works and vice versa. We tend to think of incontinence or problems with the Floor as just being related to weakness of those muscles, when, in fact, such issues have more to do with how much pressure the Floor has to support. When the pressure is too high, the Floor gives way.

How well we breathe has a direct relationship to how well the core/Floor works. Breath is the internal pump that not only supplies our bodies with oxygen, but also changes the tension level to help hold our posture as we move around. The Diaphragm, or Breather muscle, relies on the anchoring power of the Encasement as well as the spring of the Floor. The combined efforts of these muscles serve as the master controller of Pressure Mechanics. Tapping into breath is the main route toward generating core power. Ultimate breath control leads to ultimate core control.

The internal pressure system is equivalent to the hydraulics of the organs. As you know by now, organs are full of fluid and air and function much like a water balloon. This water balloon relies on its Inner Core muscle function to give the balloon shape. A healthy core system has a well-organized muscle support in which the pressure of the organ system is dynamic and equalized in all directions. With the support of the Inner Core muscles, the pressure system holds the inside of the body's volume for the Outer Core muscles to work more effectively.

Both strength and coordination are equally important in the health of the core system. However, you can't improve strength without having good coordination. You are only as strong as how well any muscle is working in and of itself as well as with others. If you can control a muscle, then you can grow it. If you don't know where the muscle is or what it does, it's hard to change it.

When you try to improve the strength and coordination of the Outer Core system without making sure that the Inner Core is working well, it always ends in Outer Core compensation. This compensation can manifest in various ways depending on the individual, but it almost always leads to a loss of internal pressure control. This leads to big problems for ladies, like back and pelvic pain, incontinence, organ prolapse, constipation, and painful sex.

The Inner Core mechanics must have the right balance of coordinated tensions to hold the volume of the pressure system and perform the movement of breathing. This tension dynamic should then be strong and capable enough to match the capabilities of the Outer Core. When these two systems are well matched, the strengthening process of the whole system is safe and healthy.

The right place to start with self-assessment is Inner Core muscle coordination. Rolling through this process not only provides insight as to how the different parts of your body are working, but it also facilitates self-awareness. Many coordination or muscle memory problems are outside of the scope of our awareness. You don't necessarily know if you aren't breathing well. Your muscle memory is what seems normal to you even if it isn't working well. You may think you know how to contract your Floor, but you might just be bearing down. You may think you can tighten your Encasement muscle, but you might just be bracing with the Six-Pack and Obliques instead.

Self-Assessment

We are going to take this process step-by-step to build your self-awareness. We begin by helping you understand how you breathe and feel what the Breather muscle is doing. Then we'll walk through the process of finding your Pelvic Floor and then your Encasement muscle. The goal is to gain awareness of how well these muscles are coordinated before they are loaded with exercise. If you have bad habits to begin with, they will only get worse with load.

Sometimes it is helpful to get a friend or partner to read the directions and self-assessment questions to you so that you can focus your attention completely on your body. Set up a table next to you with some paper and a pen. Do the check-in steps, then write down your answers to all the questions posed below.

Breath Check, in Two Parts

Quick anatomy reminder: The Breather muscle is attached all around the base of the chest bone, rib cage, and the front of the spine. The fibers of this muscle come up and attach to a central tendon, forming a dome-shaped muscle (elastic plate) that flattens and expands when it contracts.

Part One

- Position yourself on the edge of a chair in a relaxed but neutral posture (no slumping).
- Place one hand over the top part of the chest bone and the other hand at the bottom of the chest bone, covering the part where the ribs connect.

- Close your eyes and connect with where your hands are and what they are feeling.
- Take a long, slow, deep breath while staying connected with your hands.
- Repeat deep breathing for 10 repetitions as you consider these questions:

1. When you begin your inhalation, what moves first: your top hand or your bottom hand?
2. Are your shoulders lifting up as you inhale?
3. Are your shoulders lifting up along with your top hand as you are inhaling?
4. Is your bottom hand moving up and away when you begin your inhale?
5. How long is your inhalation compared to your exhalation? (Measure this by counting.)

You know your Breather muscle is working well with the function of breathing when the bottom hand leads the breath through the entire inhalation and then drops back in during exhalation. The shoulders remain quiet through the entire cycle. The length of a long inhalation should last anywhere from 4 to 7 seconds, and the exhalation phase should be even longer by another 2 to 3 seconds.

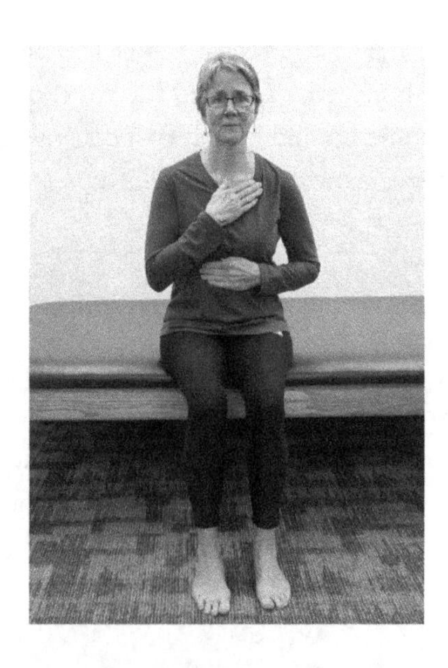

Part Two

- Remain seated in the chair with neutral posture.
- Place both hands on the sides of the lower half of your rib cage, spreading your fingers.
- Close your eyes and connect with where your hands are and what they are feeling.
- Take a long, slow, deep breath while staying connected with your hands.
- Repeat deep breath for 5 repetitions as you consider these questions:

    1. When you begin your breath, do you feel any movement in the side of your rib cage?
    2. Are your shoulders lifting up at any point in the breath cycle?
    3. Do your ribs expand and spread as you inhale?

You know your Breather muscle is working well when both hands are moving away from each other from the beginning of the breath and throughout the entire inhalation. Your hands moving away from each other indicates that the rib cage is expanding and using the full power of the entire muscle.

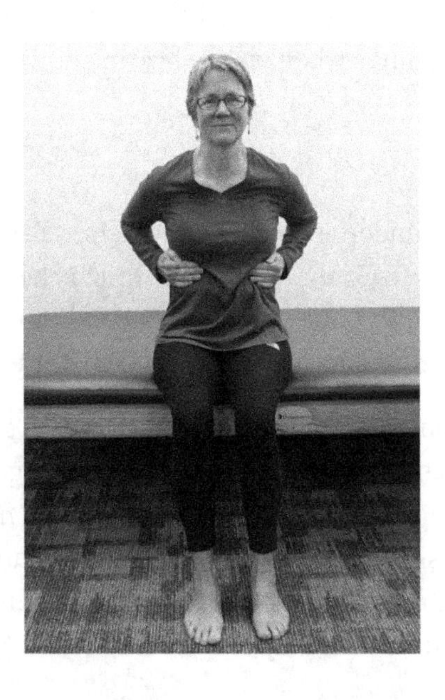

Typical Compensations That Diminish the Power of Breath

Read through the following descriptions of compensations and compare them to your answers for the exercise questions. If you are breathing in either of the following ways, you have core work to do.

Chest breathing. When the Breather muscle isn't working well, taking a deep breath can happen only by lifting the shoulders up along with the upper part of the chest. This action lifts the cage to help pull breath in, overloading the muscles of the neck and upper back, which is very hard on the heart and lungs. There is no expansion of the sides of the cage because the Breather muscle is not being used well. Typically, the length of inhalation is just a few seconds, with an even shorter exhalation.

Bearing down. This is a common action of compensation by the Breather muscle, particularly in response to pain. The muscle is pushing down on the organ balloon but not actually working to pull air into the lungs. This is the direction of muscle contraction that the Diaphragm uses when using the bathroom, especially when constipated. This downward force on the organs helps move the bowels. There is no movement of the cage under the hands when we are bearing down.

Pelvic Floor Check

Quick anatomy reminder: The Pelvic Floor muscles form a hammock shape that attaches from the tailbone through the insides of the sitz bones up to the pubic bone. This hammock-shaped muscle (elastic plate) contracts and flattens to lift the bottom of the organ balloon.

- Position yourself on the edge of a chair with good neutral posture, then slide back an inch from the edge while avoiding slumping into the back of the chair. This helps situate a better access for your hands to try to reach under the sides of your bottom. Some people have longer arms and can actually reach all the way to their sitz bones. Sometimes it is also helpful to sit on a pillow to give your hands more space. It is important to avoid slumping in an effort to extend your reach.

- Close your eyes and connect with where your hands are and what they are feeling.
- Visualize an imaginary line that begins at your tailbone and ends at your pubic bone.
- Draw muscle tension through that line as though you are pulling your tailbone and pubic bone together (the tailbone and pubic bone do not actually move, but the muscle does).
- Observe what your body does in response.

The active contraction in the Pelvic Floor feels like a light to medium lifting tension that connects from the tailbone to the pubic bone. It is common to have a greater awareness of one end or the other, especially the tailbone end. It is this kind of tension that we use to hold in gas when we're in a public place.

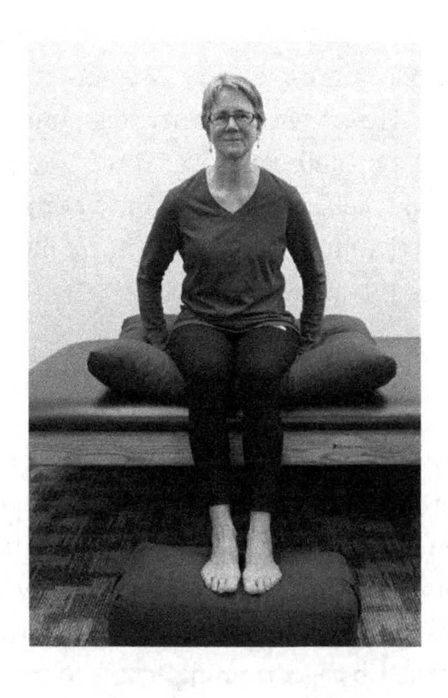

Typical Compensations That Diminish the Power of Floor Support

Read through the following descriptions of compensations and compare them to your answers for the exercise questions. If you are breathing in either of the following ways, you have core work to do.

Bearing down. This is the most common action women do when asked to perform a Pelvic Floor contraction (which you've probably heard referred to as "Kegel exercises"). They use their Diaphragm to push the organ balloon down into their Floor. This feeling of pushing down makes some women believe that it is the same as contracting and lifting. It all has to do with muscle memory. Some women start the contraction of lifting, then bear down with their Breather muscle. The muscle memory of bearing down is so ingrained that it has replaced the actual ability of the Floor to lift. It's crucial to replace this type of memory with the correct contraction technique, especially if you plan to progress into more strenuous exercise.

Butt squeezing. This is another common action we use to hold our bottoms when our Floor muscle can't. We squeeze our glutes and/or inner thigh muscles. The glutes and inner thigh muscles have no direct attachment to the Floor and can never directly support the bladder, vagina, or anus. If you feel any muscles contracting in the area of your butt or inner thighs, then it is likely that you are not performing a contraction of the Pelvic Floor.

Encasement Muscle Check, in Three Parts

Quick anatomy reminder: The Encasement muscle is quite large, with a lot of points of attachment. The lower part attaches from the sides of the lower lumbar spine, all along the top sides of the bones of the pelvis, running across to meet in the middle under the belly button. The upper half of the muscles attach from the side of the upper lumbar spine all along the edges of the rib cage, running across to meet in the middle at and above the belly button. The tension of the Encasement is partnered with both of its plate muscles (the Breather and the Floor muscles) and needs to be assessed in relationship to both ends, as well as to its own ability to hold power.

Part One

- Position yourself on the edge of a chair with erect, neutral posture.
- Cover your lower belly with the palms of both hands, above the pubic bone and below the belly button.
- Close your eyes and connect with where your hands are and what they are feeling.
- Perform a Pelvic Floor contraction in which you are connecting the tailbone and the pubic bone with the tension that lifts up your Floor.

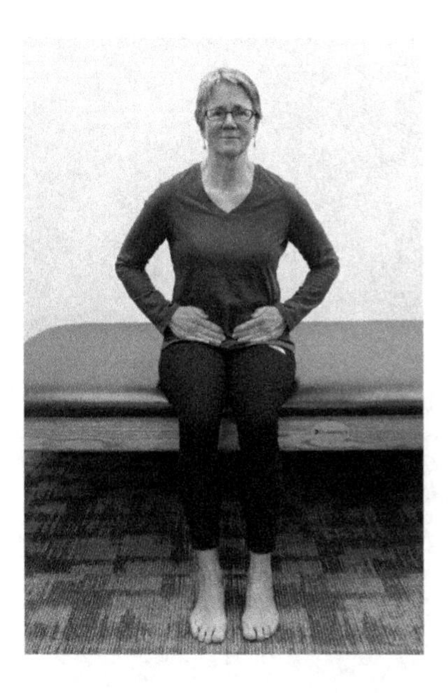

The lower half of the Encasement muscle responds to the Floor muscle contraction with a contraction of its own. These two muscles share a muscle memory of working together. As you contract your Pelvic Floor, tune in to the light tension of the lower half of the Encasement muscle that occurs naturally with the Floor. If you are unable to accurately perform a Pelvic Floor contraction, then you will not be able to tune in to this tension relationship between the Floor and the Encasement.

Part Two

- Position yourself on the edge of a chair with erect, neutral posture.
- Cover your upper belly at the belly button with the palm of one hand, and place the other hand just above that but below the rib cage.
- Close your eyes and connect with where your hands are and what they are feeling.
- Take a long, slow, deep breath while staying connected with your hands.
- Repeat deep breath for 3 cycles.

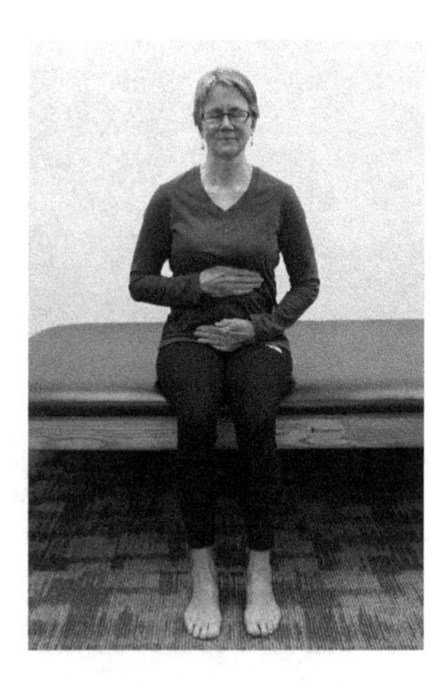

The action of breath begins with an expansion around the full circle of the base of the rib cage. This expansion of the cage extends into the abdomen all the way down to the pelvis. The length of inhaled breath in is usually 4 to 7 seconds, and the abdomen and cage return to their start position with exhaled breath lasting 6 to 8 seconds. If you are compensating with a chest breathing pattern, then you will be unable to feel that expansion that descends from the base of the cage through the abdomen all the way into the pelvis.

Part Three

- Position yourself on the edge of a chair with erect, neutral posture.
- Cover your lower belly above the pubic bone and below the belly button with the palms of both hands.
- Close your eyes and connect with where your hands are and what they are feeling.
- Purse your lips and blow as though you are blowing through a straw. Continue to blow for as long as you can, monitoring the tensions of your belly.
- Notice the tension of the Encasement muscle as it draws in and almost shrink-wraps the organ balloon. Hold that tension and resume normal breath rhythm. Relax that tension and then see if you can actively recover it.

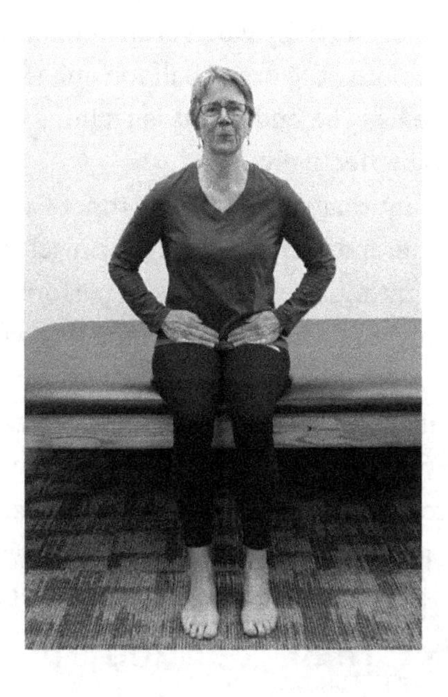

The fiber direction of the Encasement muscle is horizontal; therefore, when we actively engage this muscle, it will rein in the entire wall of muscle, feeling almost like a shrink-wrapping of the waist. This is a different feeling than that of the other muscles of the abdominal wall. The Encasement muscle is primary in helping force air up through the mouth, so when you blow through a straw, you will feel that muscle during the last few seconds of exhaling. Then you test your ability to actively engage the muscle by actively contracting it while you breathe normally.

Typical Compensations That Diminish the Power of Encasement Muscle Support

The Six-Pack and the Obliques have fiber directions that are vertical in nature, whereas the Encasement muscle's direction is horizontal. When the vertical muscles are compensating for the Encasement, there is a lot of tension that pulls the front of the rib cage downward toward the pelvis. This vertical tension causes a doming effect or a pooch in the belly. This is key to monitor while doing any core exercise. If there is doming or pooching of the belly when crunching or planking, then the Encasement is not holding the organ balloon and the bones effectively, which causes problems. The end result is training both the Outer and Inner Core muscles ineffectively.

It is very important that you start your Inner Core assessment with looking at the Breather muscle and the Floor muscle before the Encasement. The Encasement muscle's abilities to perform are so linked with its plates that you might mistake what's happening with it. The inability to actively contract the Floor or breathe properly will make things feel different. For instance, if you are doing a lot of bearing down with a Floor contraction or exhale action, the Encasement muscle will look and feel very different. It is easy to mistake an activation of the vertical muscles (Six-Pack and Obliques) with a bearing down.

Bringing a Picture of Your Body Together

You now know where your Breather, Encasement, and Floor muscles are and how they are working. If your self-assessment identified any issues or problems, they must be addressed before moving forward into the more common core strengthening exercise approaches. It is not worth the many negative consequences that can occur when you try to skip coordinating your Inner Core and rush into strength training.

The next four chapters will walk you through an exercise progression designed to restore the activation patterns of normal muscle memory of each Inner Core muscle, as well as the process of integrating these new memories into activities of daily living.

CHAPTER 14

Core Focus Exercise

One of the toughest parts of the rehabilitation process is pausing to get focused with awareness. Some people do not have a good sense of where their body parts are and are reluctant to take the time to find them. There is also a lot of frustration in finding a muscle activation when its muscle memory has been changed. It can be so frustrating that many decide it can't be done, and they just move on and do the best they can.

You may believe that there is no way something could be wrong with your breathing because, surely, you would notice that . . . right? Believe it or not, breath holding is a very popular strategy for cheating your way through an exercise. It's not even something that most people are aware they are doing, and there are a lot of things that cause people to change the way they breathe. There is only one way to get it back. Practice and awareness!

Reconnecting your Inner Core begins with restoring your coordinative control of all three inner core muscles. It might be worth rereading chapter 4 to remind yourself of the differences in training coordination versus strengthening exercise. These concepts are frequently misunderstood and contribute to many mistakes in core training. Restoring the coordinative control and muscle memory must happen before actual strengthening can be meaningful—otherwise you are just training compensation.

All three muscles of the Inner Core are multitaskers. In other words, they perform multiple actions at the same time. The Breather Muscle performs the action of breath and simultaneously generates different levels of tension to hold posture of the bones. The Encasement muscle assists in the exhale phase of breath while supporting the bones posturally. The Floor muscle maintains continence as well as assisting the Encasement muscle. Core Focus exercises are where we start to recover active control of all the different tasks these muscles are responsible for.

Keys to Success for Inner Core Training

- Start from the beginning and learn to coordinate the muscles and breath.
- Begin slowly so that you can process what you are feeling.
- Practice the contraction.
- Practice the contraction intensity levels.
- Practice the contraction hold times.
- Practice mixing up the different intensities and the different hold times.
- Change positions and start all over.

Breather Muscle

- Get comfortable lying on your back with a small pillow under your head and a bigger pillow under your knees. Rest one hand on your lower belly and the other one at the base of the front of the rib cage.

- Focus your awareness on long, slow, deep breaths in which your hands can feel the expansion of breath from the base of the cage. This expansion will travel throughout the belly into the pelvis. Sometimes it is nice to have a bag of dry beans resting under the top hand at the base of the rib cage. The weight helps orient the brain to better coordinate breath.

- Count how long you can lengthen both the inhale and exhale phases. Compare this to what feels like your normal length of breath.

- Repeat for 10 long, slow, deep breaths, then compare again to what your regular breath rhythm feels like.

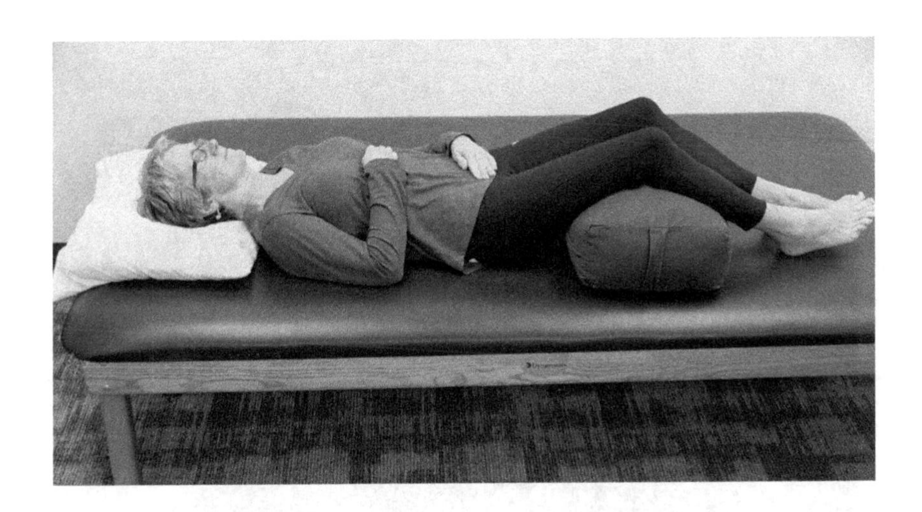

Floor Muscle

- Remain resting comfortably on your back with your head and knees supported. Place both of your hands over the bones of the pelvis.
- Close your eyes and imagine a line from the tailbone connecting to the pubic bone. Put tension through this line, as though you are trying to draw your tailbone and pubic bone together. You will feel a sense of lift as the muscle contracts.
- Hold the contraction, then slowly relax. Repeat 10 times.
- Be aware of gripping tension from your Gluteus (butt) or inner thigh muscles. These are not a part of the Floor muscle function but are called upon to cheat. Keep these muscles separate from the tension of lifting the Floor.
- Hold awareness of your breath and the possibility of bearing down. If you feel yourself pushing from your Breather muscle, as though you are doing a bowel motion, then you are not correctly activating the Floor muscle.
- As you repeat the contraction of the Floor, start to notice a tension across the lower belly, as though your belly is flattening and drawing in. That is your Encasement muscle, which automatically activates when you use your Floor muscle.

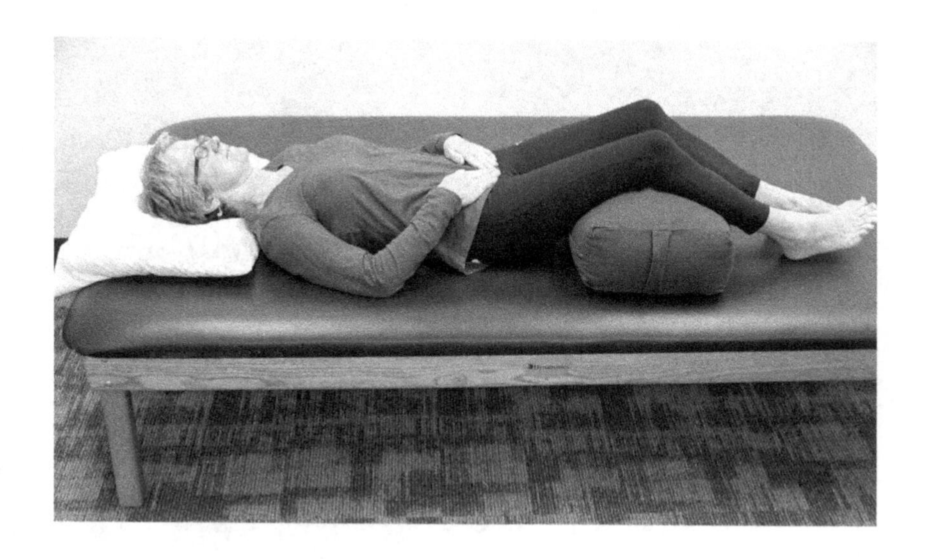

Encasement Muscle

It's a little bit more challenging to find and activate the tension of the Encasement because this muscle lives under the Six-Pack and the Obliques. It is easy to mistake the tension of the Encasement for the tension of the other muscles. It's important to remember that the Encasement muscle fibers run horizontally from one bone of the pelvis that goes straight across to the other bone. We can recover the ability to focus tension of activation by using resistance with the exhale phase of breath with a trick called "blow through a straw" as well as the tension from a Floor contraction.

- Start by remaining resting comfortably on your back with your head and knees supported and both of your hands over the bones of the pelvis.
- Purse your lips and blow as though you are blowing through a straw. Hold the rate of blowing steady and make it last as long as you can. As you reach the end of your exhale, you will notice that flattening tension, as though your belly is being shrink-wrapped. That is the tension of the Encasement muscle.

- Hold that tension and resume a regular breath.
- Slightly relax that tension, then ramp it back up and hold.
- Let everything completely relax, then try to resume that same tension of the same muscle.
- Test to see if you've got the right tension with a recheck using blow through a straw.
- Practice until you can actively put tension through the Encasement muscle without using the blow-through-a-straw trick.

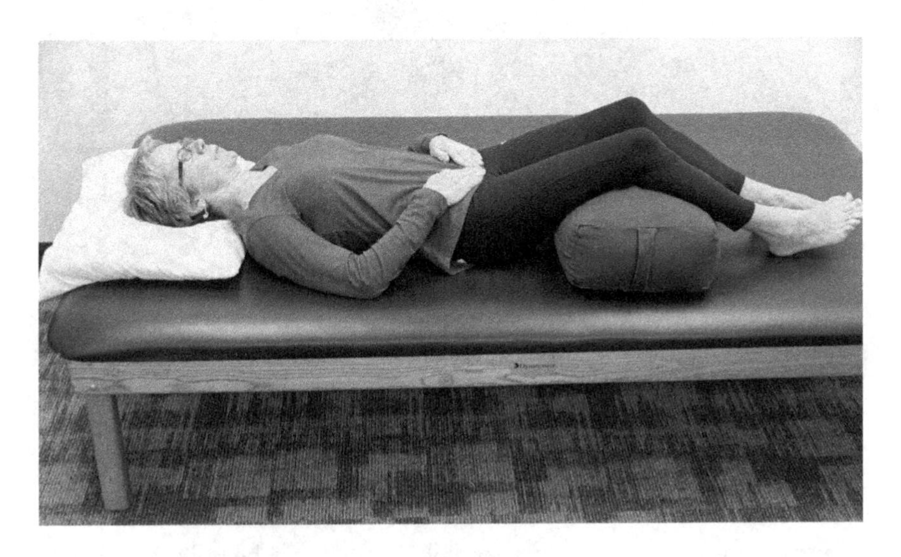

Combine the Three

- Remain resting comfortably on your back with your head and knees supported and both of your hands over the bones of the pelvis.
- Begin with the expansion of a nice, long inhale, with that expansion reaching into the Floor. As you begin your exhale, add tension to the Encasement and the Floor muscles.
- Repeat this cycle 5 times.

- Repeat the inhale expansion again, but now vary the intensity of the exhale tension by alternating between the Encasement and the Floor. Try one breath with focused activation on the Encasement. With the next breath, focus activation intensity on the Floor.
- Repeat and alternate for 6 cycles.

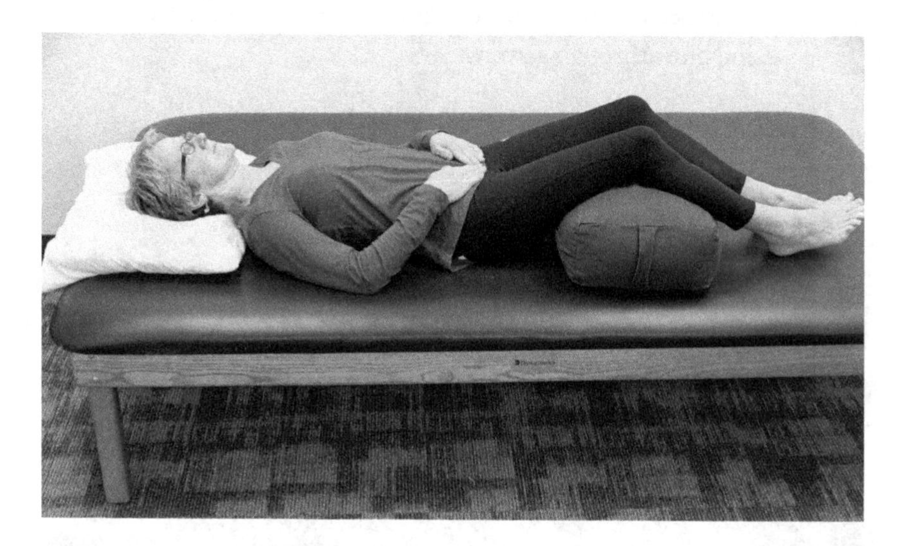

Focused Practice of Encasement and Floor Coordination

Normal motion and activities require that these muscles alter tension levels regardless of what stage the breath cycle is in. Tension levels can vary from low to medium to high. You should be able to perform a sustained low tension that you can quickly ramp in and out of all the other levels of tension. It helps to imagine each muscle with a dial that directs the tension level. We will be practicing changing the tension levels of the Floor and the Encasement in a step-by-step order as well as randomly.

- Start by remaining resting comfortably on your back with your head and knees supported and both of your hands over the bones of the pelvis.

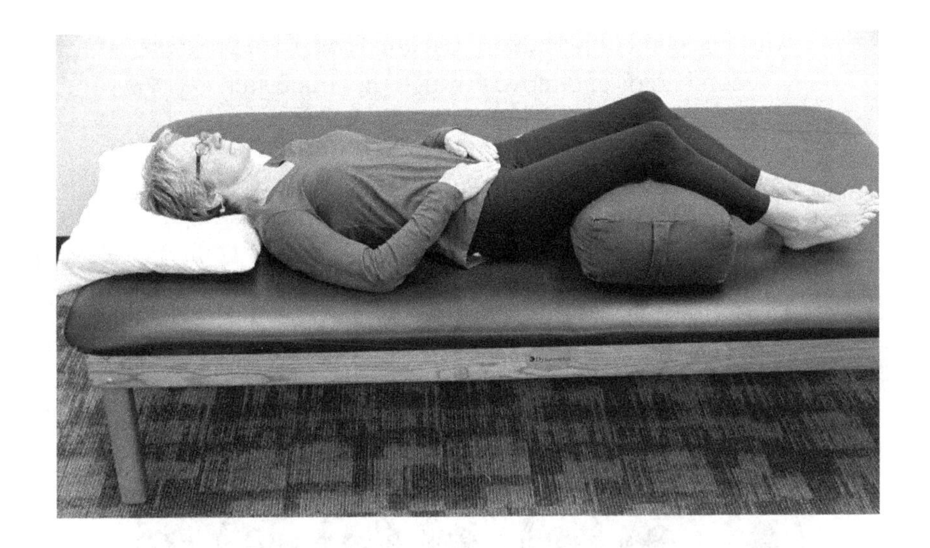

- Begin with the Floor tension. Connect the tailbone and pubic bone, then lift the Floor with the lowest tension possible (tension level 1). Hold this tension and then ratchet it up to a slightly higher tension (tension level 2). Now ratchet it up to the next level of tension possible (tension level 3). Finish this drill with increasing the tension to its highest level (tension level 4). Be careful not to muscle the tension up with your Six-Pack or Oblique muscles.
- Stairstep the tension levels (that is, proceed in 1-2-3-4-3-2-1 order), holding each level for 5 seconds each. Repeat stairstep tension, moving up and down through each level as fast as you can.

Tension Dials

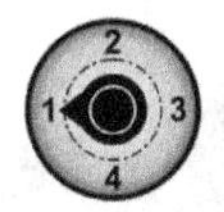

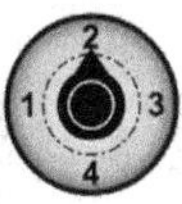

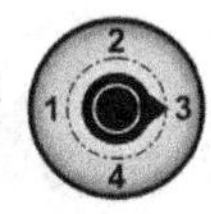

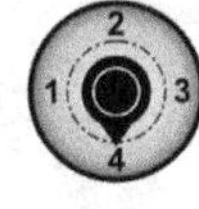

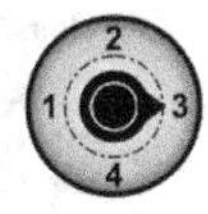

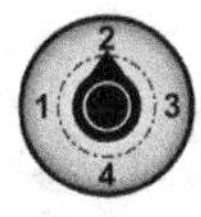

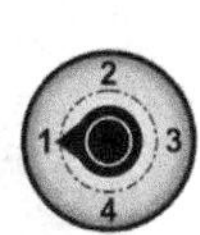

- It is important to have the ability to alternate between all levels of tension in a random manner mostly because that is the way these tensions function in all our life activities. Here are some suggestions for drill practice. You can begin with 5-second holds at each tension level, then progress to 1-second holds and move through the drill faster.

- Find and activate the tension of the Encasement. Hold the lowest tension possible (level 1), then ramp it up to level 2, level 3, and then finally level 4.

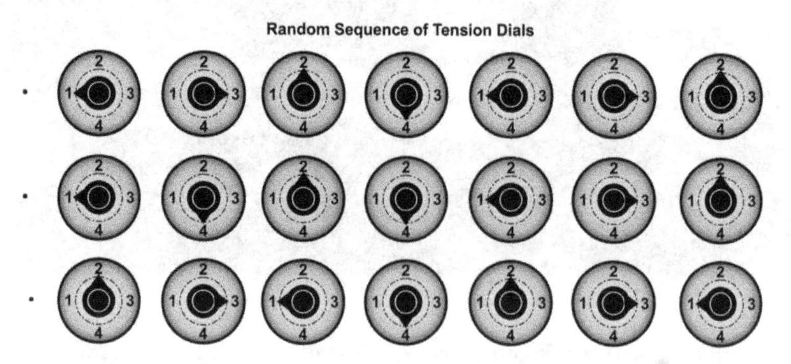

- Return to stairstepping the tension levels like this: 1-2-3-2-1. Begin each step of tension and hold for 5 seconds before moving to the next step. Repeat and increase the speed of the steps.

Tension Dials

- The final step for focused practice is to alternate between all of the different tension levels randomly. Here are some suggestions for practicing alternation of varying tension levels:

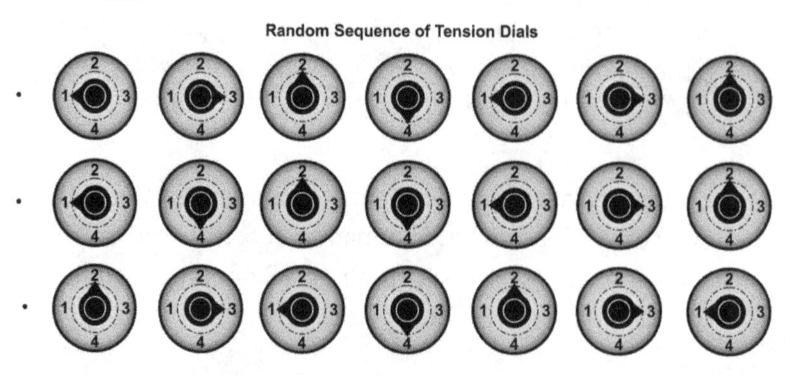

CHAPTER 15

Core Gravity Exercise

When you feel confident that you can consistently perform the Core Focus exercises, then it is time to challenge your coordination in other positions. Many women prefer to skip this stage of exercise because it is deceptively challenging. These are called Core Gravity exercises because your body is upright and gravity is loading your bones and muscles. These exercises are deceptive because you will be doing the same basic activities, but in a sitting and/or standing position.

Most people find at least one of these exercises extremely difficult because it just doesn't feel the same in an upright position compared to lying down. In fact, many become so frustrated that they skip it altogether. The unfortunate result of this is the muscle memory that is necessary for restoring full core coordination is never recovered. It is important to stay on track with core coordination recovery by mastering each activity in order.

I recommend beginning with the Core Gravity exercise in a sitting position. There is a lot for your brain to pay attention to and sitting position allows your brain to just focus on everything between the head and pelvis. There is a range of ideal positioning, with the goal being an even weight distribution of the head over the cage over the pelvis. It is this range of neutral that you want to practice Core Gravity exercise.

You will want to sit on the edge of a chair with both your feet on the floor. Close your eyes so you can bring awareness to how you are distributing the weight of your bones as well as how your muscles are working. Ask yourself these questions:

- Are you sitting over both of your sitz bones evenly?
- Are you loading one side more heavily than the other?
- Are you rocked back onto your tailbone or forward on your pubic bone?

Check in with how your rib cage orients over your pelvis.

- Do you feel like you are arching your back with the weight of your cage hanging in front of your pelvis?
- Is the front of your chest slumped down?
- How relaxed are your shoulders?

Spend some time rocking the weight of the pelvis side to side and front to back until you feel you have a neutral distribution of weight. Arch and slump your back until you find the sense of balancing your cage over your pelvis. Test out how relaxed your shoulders are by taking a big deep breath. After you accomplish this, open your eyes and make note of where you are. Now you are ready for Core Gravity exercise.

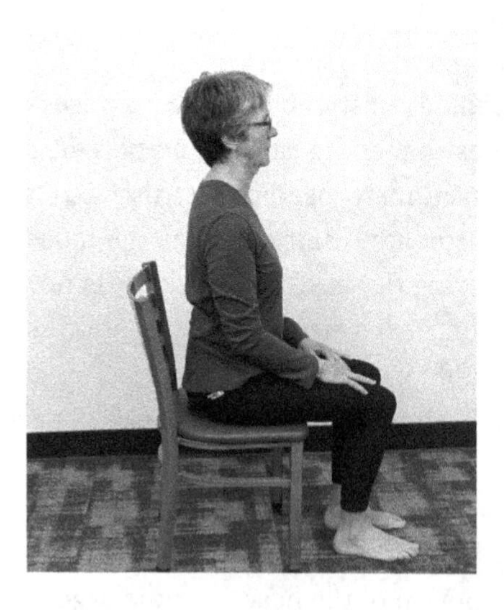

Breather Muscle

- Sit at the edge of a chair in neutral position, as described previously, resting both hands over the sides of your pelvic bones.

- Place one hand on your lower belly and the other hand at the base of your rib cage in the front.
- Focus on taking long, slow, deep breaths in which your hands can feel the expansion of breath from the base of the cage. This expansion will travel throughout the belly into the pelvis.
- Count how long you can lengthen both the inhale and exhale phases. Compare this to what feels like your normal length of breath.
- Repeat for 10 long, slow, deep breaths, then compare again to what your regular breath rhythm feels like.

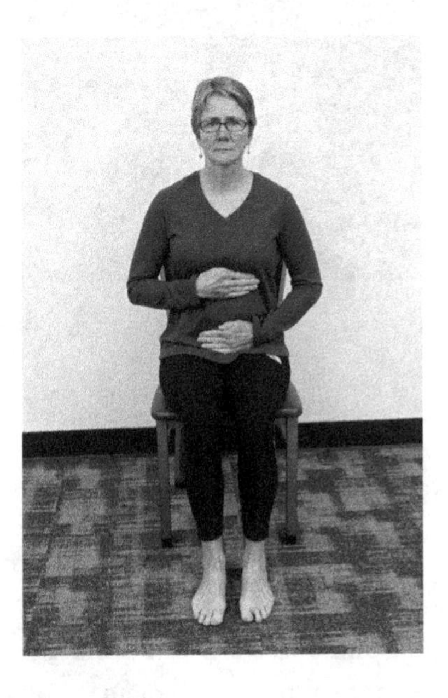

- Change the placement of your hands to the sides of your cage. Take a long, slow, deep breath and note the rib cage expanding into your hands as you breathe.

- Keeping this hand placement, repeat for another 10 long, slow, deep breaths, then compare again to what your regular breath rhythm feels like.

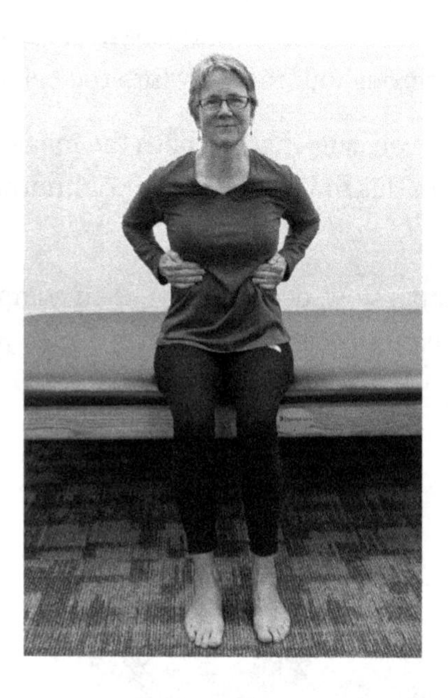

Floor Muscle

- Sit at the edge of a chair in neutral position, resting both hands over the sides of your pelvic bones.
- Close your eyes and imagine a line from the tailbone connecting to the pubic bone. Put tension through this line, as though you are trying to draw your tailbone and pubic bone together. You should feel a sense of lift as the muscle contracts.
- Hold the contraction, then slowly relax. Repeat 10 times.
- Be aware of gripping tension from your glutes and/or inner thigh muscles. Also make note of the tension of the Six-Pack and Oblique muscles where they attach at the base of the cage.
- Hold awareness of your breath and the possibility of bearing down. If you feel yourself pushing from your Breather muscle as though

you are doing a bowel motion, then you are not correctly activating the Floor muscle.

- As you repeat the contraction of the Floor, you will start to notice a tension across the lower belly as though your belly is flattening and drawing in. That is your Encasement muscle working in tandem with the Floor.

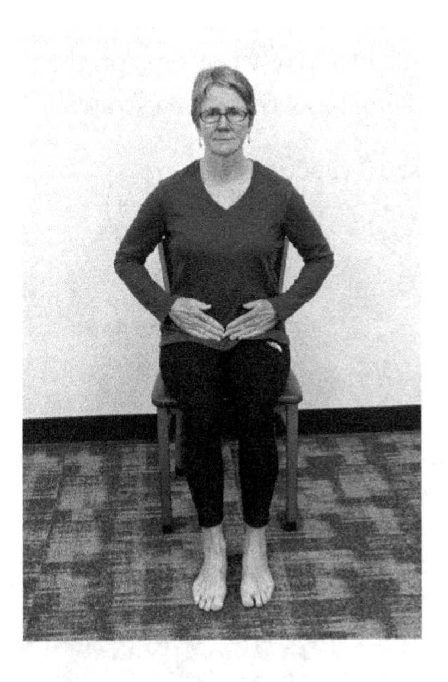

Encasement Muscle

- Sit at the edge of a chair in neutral position, resting both hands over the sides of your pelvic bones.
- Find the tension of the Encasement muscle with the blow-through-a-straw trick. Purse your lips and blow as though you are blowing through a straw. Hold the rate of blowing steady and make it last as long as you can. As you reach the end of your exhale, you will notice that flattening tension, as though your belly is being shrink-wrapped around and in. That is the tension of the Encasement muscle.

- Hold that tension and resume a regular breath.
- Slightly relax that tension, then ramp it back up and hold.
- Let everything completely relax, then try to resume that same tension of the same muscle.
- Test to see if you've got the right tension by rechecking with the blow-through-a-straw trick.
- Practice until you can actively put tension through the Encasement muscle without using blow through a straw.
- Repeat for at least 10 repetitions.

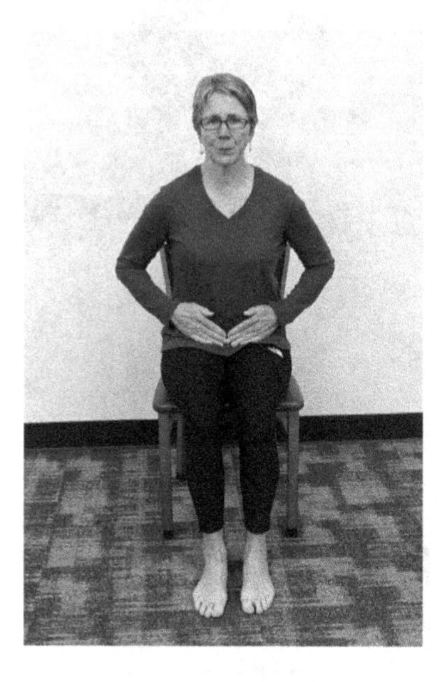

Combining the Three

- Sit at the edge of a chair in neutral position, resting both hands over the sides of your pelvic bones.
- Begin with the expansion created by a nice, long inhale, with that expansion reaching into the Floor. As you begin your exhale, add tension to the Encasement and the Floor muscles.

- Repeat this cycle 5 times.
- Repeat the inhale expansion again, but vary the intensity of the exhale tension by alternating between the Encasement and the Floor. Try one breath with focused activation on the Encasement. With the next breath, focus activation intensity on the Floor.
- Repeat and alternate for 6 cycles.

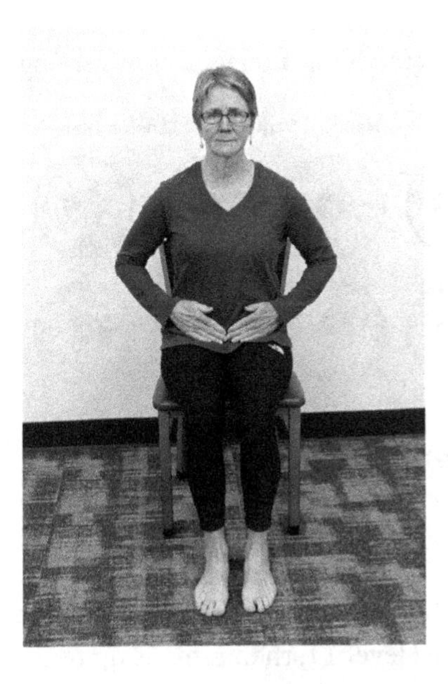

Focused Practice of Encasement and Floor Coordination

- Sit at the edge of a chair in neutral position, resting both hands over the sides of your pelvic bones.
- Begin with the Floor tension. Connect the tailbone and pubic bone, then lift the Floor with the lowest tension possible (tension level 1). Hold this tension and then ratchet it up to a slightly higher tension (tension level 2). Now increase the tension another notch (tension level 3) and then up to the highest tension possible (tension level 4).

- Stairstep the tension levels in 1-2-3-4-3-2-1 order, holding each level for 5 seconds. Repeat stairstep tension, moving up and down each level as fast as you can.

Tension Dials

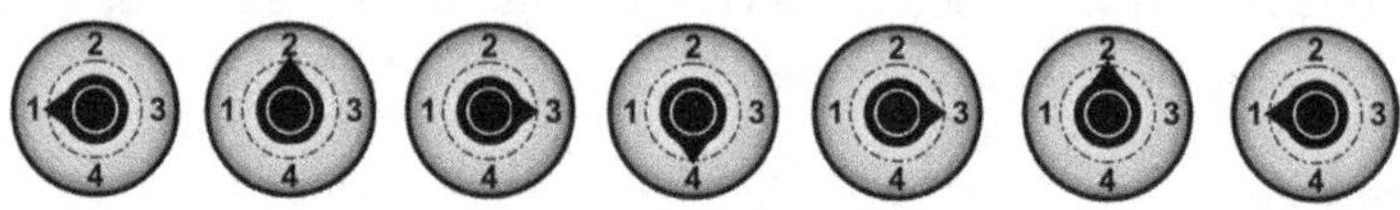

- Suggestions for practicing alternation of varying tension levels:

Random Sequence of Tension Dials

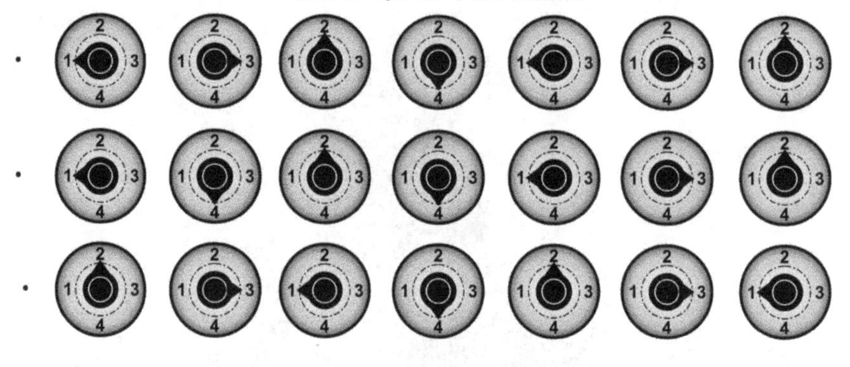

- Find and activate the tension of the Encasement. Hold the lowest tension possible (level 1), then ramp it up to level 2, then level 3 and finally level 4.
- Return to stairstepping the tension levels thusly: 1-2-3-4-3-2-1. Begin each step of tension and hold for 5 seconds before moving to the next step. Repeat and increase the speed of the steps.

Tension Dials

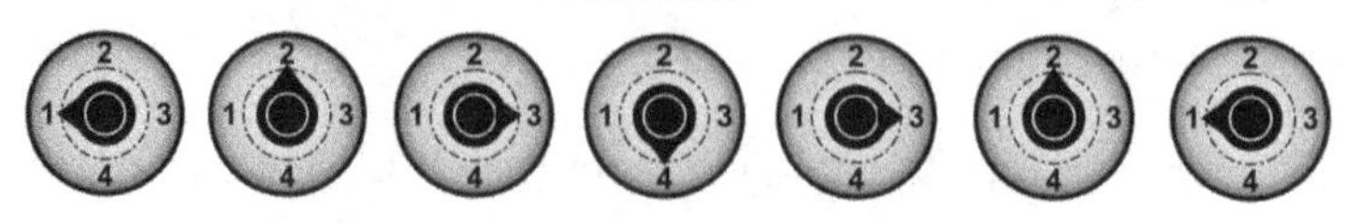

- Suggestions for practicing alternation of varying tension levels:

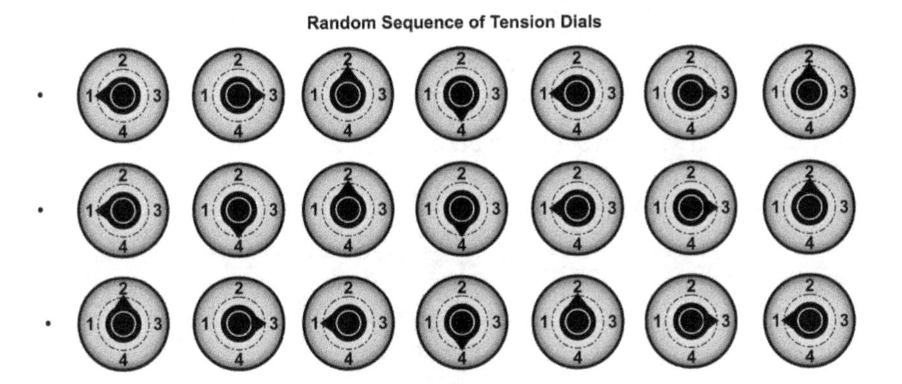

Begin Resisted Breath

Resisting breath is basically pulling air in through an aperture or hole that resists the flow of air. To reduce the resistance of airflow and make it easier, you can make this hole bigger. To increase the resistance to airflow, you make this hole smaller, which makes it more challenging to pull air in and push air out. Resistance with pulling air in loads and works the Diaphragm. Resistance with flowing air out works the Encasement and Floor muscles.

You can find a resisted breath device fairly easily online for a reasonable price. Doing a search for the words "breathing training devices" should yield you different options. Some therapy exercise approaches use a balloon to practice resisted breath. Whereas this might be interesting to try, the balloon can only resist the ability to blow air and does not offer a steady, sustained resistance. You can also purse your lips to resist airflow both ways, but it can become awkward and inconsistent.

- Start by sitting at the edge of a chair in neutral position, resting both hands over the sides of your pelvic bones.

- Place the device in your mouth and begin with the expansion of a nice, long inhale, pulling in air through the device rather than through your nose. This expansion should reach into the Floor. As you blow through the device and begin your exhale, focus tension on the Encasement and Floor muscles to complete the full exhalation.

- Maintain a slow, steady pace through the full excursion of inhale and exhale. Resist the desire to flex into it and muscle your way through the breath.
- Repeat this cycle 20 times.

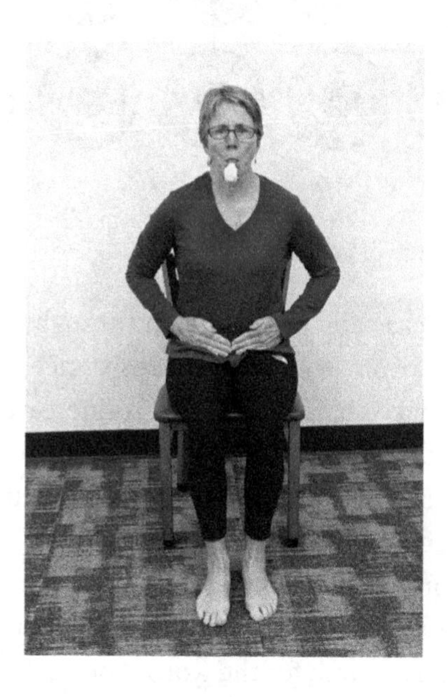

After you feel confident in your ability to coordinate all of these different muscle contractions and breath work exercises in sitting position, it's time to further challenge things by standing. Basically, we will be going through the same lineup of activities we did while sitting, ending with practicing resisted breath.

Again, there's a proper stance to take that will apply throughout this whole round of exercises. It begins by pulling your awareness to your feet as you stand. Do you have an equal amount of weight on both feet? Maintain a neutral knee over the top of each foot. Is your pelvis swayed forward in front of your feet, or is it tucked back behind your feet? Once you have balanced your pelvis over your feet, check in with your rib cage. Is it arched forward over the pelvis, or is it slumped behind the pelvis?

Breather Muscle

- Stand with awareness of your posture, as described above, resting both hands over the sides of your pelvic bones.
- Place one hand on your lower belly and the other hand at the base of your rib cage in the front.
- Focus your awareness on long, slow, deep breaths in which your hands can feel the expansion of breath from the base of the cage. This expansion will travel throughout the belly into the pelvis.
- Count how long you can lengthen both the inhale and exhale phases. Compare this to what feels like your normal length of breath.
- Repeat for 10 long, slow, deep breaths, then compare again to what your regular breath rhythm feels like.
- Change the placement of your hands to the sides of your cage. Take a long, slow, deep breath and note the rib cage expanding into your hands as you breathe.
- Keeping this hand placement, repeat for another 10 long, slow, deep breaths, then compare again to what your regular breath rhythm feels like.

Floor Muscle

- Stand with awareness of your posture, resting both hands over the sides of your pelvic bones.
- Close your eyes and imagine a line from the tailbone connecting to the pubic bone. Put tension through this line, as though you are trying to draw your tailbone and pubic bone together. You should feel a sense of lift as the muscle contracts.
- Hold the contraction, then slowly relax. Repeat 10 times.

- Be aware of gripping tension from your glutes and/or inner thigh muscles. Also make note of the tension of the Six-Pack and Oblique muscles where they attach at the base of the cage.
- Hold awareness of your breath and the possibility of bearing down. If you feel yourself pushing from your Breather muscle as though you are doing a bowel motion, then you are not correctly activating the Floor muscle.
- As you repeat the contraction of the Floor, start to notice a tension across the lower belly, as though your belly is flattening and drawing in. That is your Encasement muscle working in tandem with the Floor.

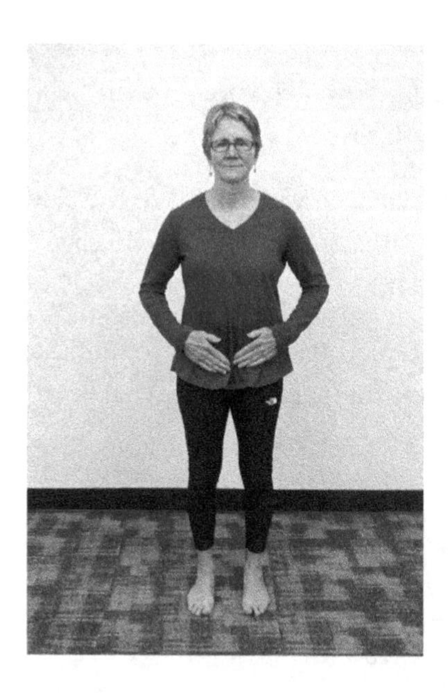

Encasement Muscle

- Stand with awareness of your posture, resting both hands over the sides of your pelvic bones.
- Find the tension of the Encasement muscle by pursing your lips and blowing as you would through a straw. Hold the rate of

blowing steady and make it last as long as you can. As you reach the end of your exhale, you will notice that flattening tension, as though your belly is being shrink-wrapped around and in. That is the tension of the Encasement muscle.

- Hold that tension and resume a regular breath.
- Slightly relax that tension, then ramp it back up and hold.
- Let everything completely relax, then try to resume that same tension of the same muscle.
- Test to see if you've got the right tension by rechecking with blow through a straw.
- Practice until you can actively put tension through the Encasement muscle without using the blow-through-a-straw trick.
- Repeat at least 10 times.

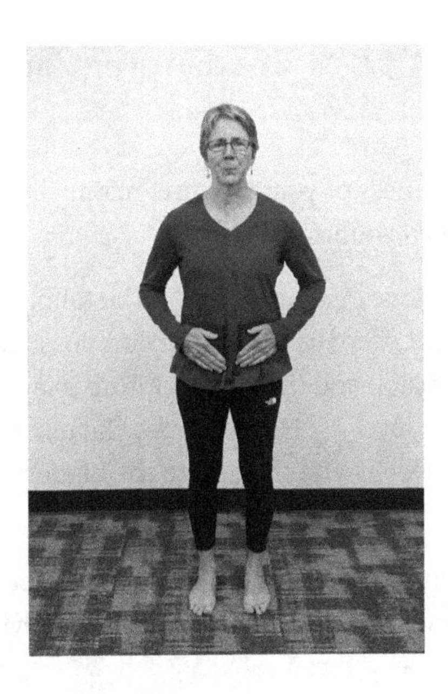

Combining the Three

- Stand with awareness of your posture, as described in the preceding exercises, resting both hands over the sides of your pelvic bones.
- Begin with the expansion created by a nice, long inhale, with that expansion reaching into the Floor. As you begin your exhale, add tension to the Encasement and the Floor muscles.
- Repeat this cycle 5 times.
- Now repeat the inhale expansion, but vary the intensity of the exhale tension by alternating between the Encasement and the Floor. Try one breath with focused activation on the Encasement. With the next breath, focus activation intensity on the Floor.
- Repeat and alternate for 6 cycles.

Focused Practice of Encasement and Floor Coordination

- Stand with awareness of your posture, resting both hands over the sides of your pelvic bones.
- Begin with the Floor tension. Connect the tailbone and pubic bone, then lift the Floor with the lowest tension possible (tension level 1). Hold this tension and then ratchet it up to a slightly higher tension (tension level 2). Now increase the tension to the next level (tension level 3) and then up to the highest tension possible (tension level 4).
- Stairstep the tension levels in 1-2-3-4-3-2-1 order, holding each level for 5 seconds. Repeat stairstep tension, moving up and down each level as fast as you can.

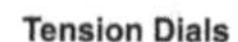

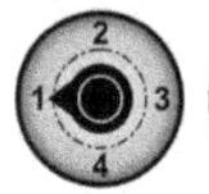

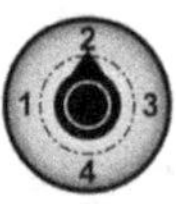

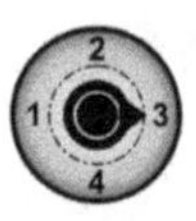

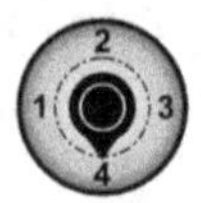

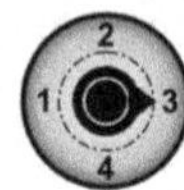

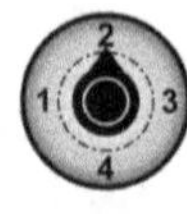

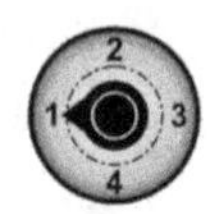

- Suggestions for practicing alternation of varying tension levels:

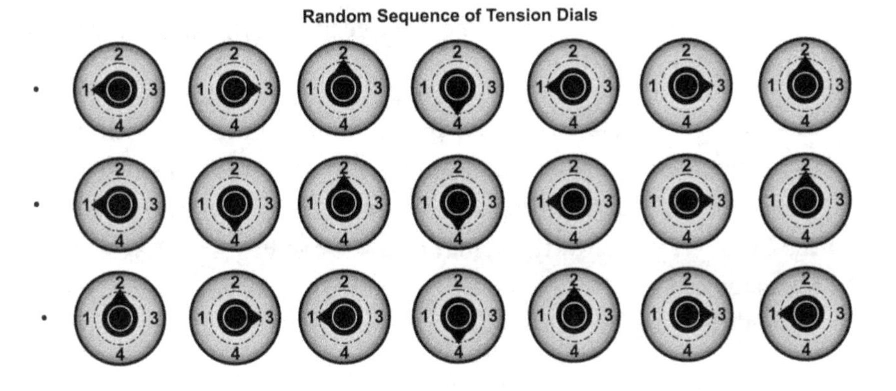

- Find and activate the tension of the Encasement. Hold the lowest tension possible (level 1), then ramp it up to level 2, then level 3 and finally level 4.
- Return to stairstepping the tension levels thusly: 1-2-3-4-3-2-1. Begin each step of tension and hold for 5 seconds before moving to the next step. Repeat and increase the speed of the steps.

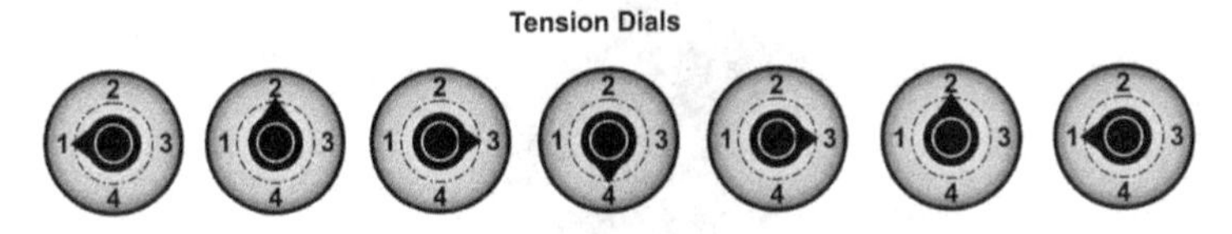

- Suggestions for practicing alternation of varying tension levels:

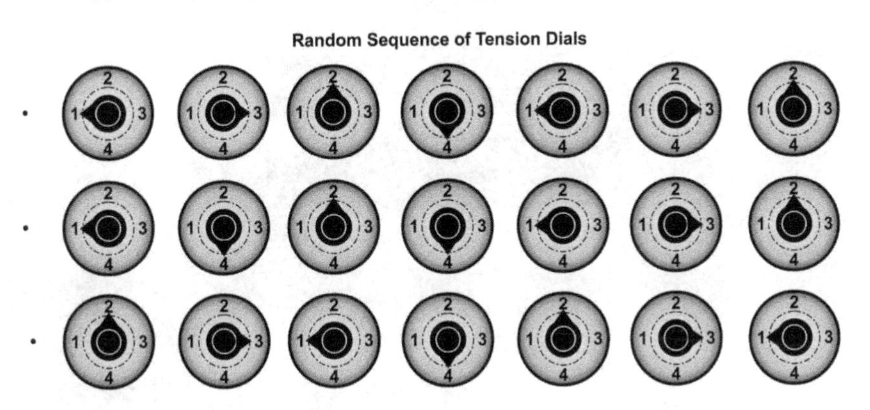

Begin Resisted Breath

- Stand with awareness of your posture, resting both hands over the sides of your pelvic bones.
- Place the resisted breath device in your mouth and begin with the expansion of a nice, long inhale, pulling in air through the device rather than through your nose. This expansion should reach into the Floor. As you blow through the device and begin your exhale, focus tension on the Encasement and Floor muscles to complete the full exhalation.
- Maintain a slow, steady pace through the full excursion of inhale and exhale. Resist the desire to flex into it and muscle your way through the breath.
- Repeat this cycle 20 times.

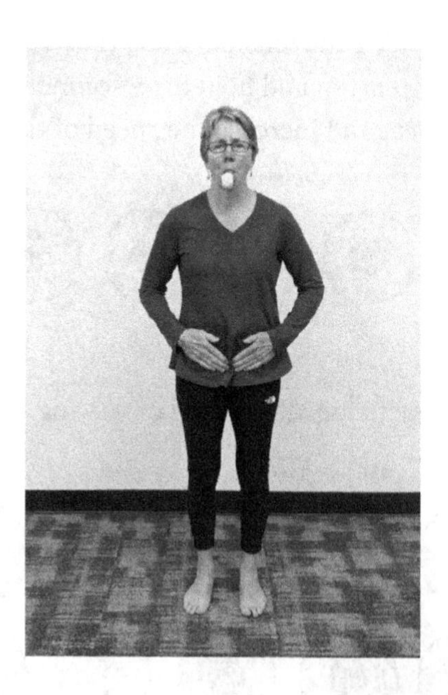

CHAPTER 16

Core Function Exercises

Once you have mastered the complete range of tension possibilities of all the Inner Core muscles in all posture positions, it is time to incorporate these tensions with movement. Core Function exercises are movement drills that focus on building the right core tension with movement. It is all too easy to fall back on old patterns of breath holding and other compensatory strategies when we are challenged with activities that require weight or exertion. Building movement habits that incorporate breath, optimal alignment, and the right level of muscle tension is key for the best exercise outcome.

Sitting Stick Lift

- Find a pole that is at least 3 feet long. Position yourself seated on the edge of a chair with your weight equally distributed on both sitz bones and your rib cage centered over your pelvis. Hold the pole out with both arms straight and palms down.
- Initiate the lift of the stick simultaneously with inhalation and lower the stick with exhalation. The technique of the activity is to coordinate the lifting with inhalation and the lowering of the stick with exhalation.
- Be mindful of your alignment. There is a tendency to slump when lowering the stick. It's okay to feel a slight sway as you lift and lower.
- You can progress this activity by adding weights to the stick or by replacing the stick with handheld weights.

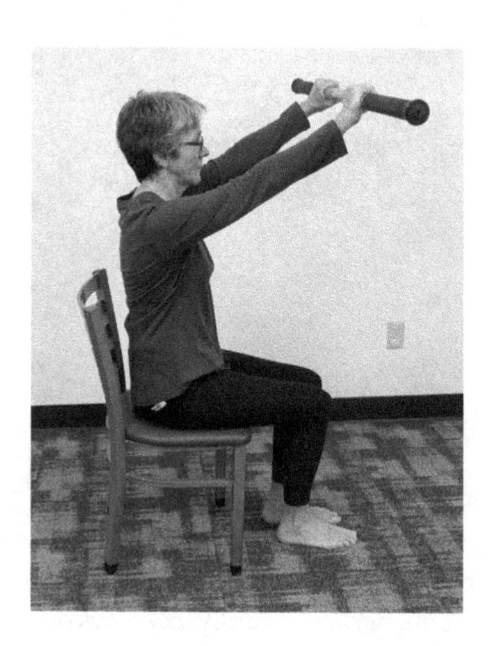

Sitting Rotation

- Position yourself seated on the edge of a chair with your weight equally distributed on both sitz bones and your rib cage centered over your pelvis. Place both hands on the sides of the rib cage.
- Coordinate inhalation with moving into rotation. Return to neutral with exhalation. Inhale to rotate right, exhale to return to center. Inhale to rotate left, exhale to return to center.
- Awareness should focus on the expansion of the cage as you twist your body, as well as on remaining centered over the pelvis.
- You can progress this activity by using the resisted breath device and/or by pulling an exercise band during rotation.

Sit to Stand

- Position yourself seated on the edge of a chair with your weight equally distributed on both sitz bones and your rib cage centered over your pelvis. Plant your feet more than shoulder width apart.

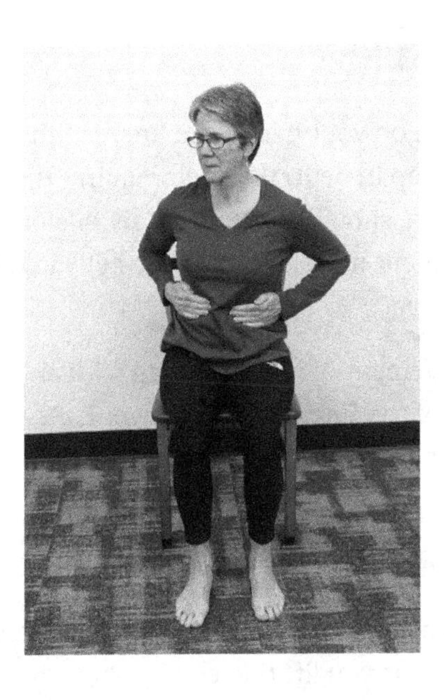

- Coordinate exhaling and ramp the tension of the Encasement and the Floor up to level 2 as you tip forward to lift your hips off the chair. Once you are standing, drop the tension back to level 1. Exhale and ramp tension up to level 2 to return to sitting.
- It's important to remember to coordinate the tension within the movement pattern, as well as to hinge at the hips to return to sitting.

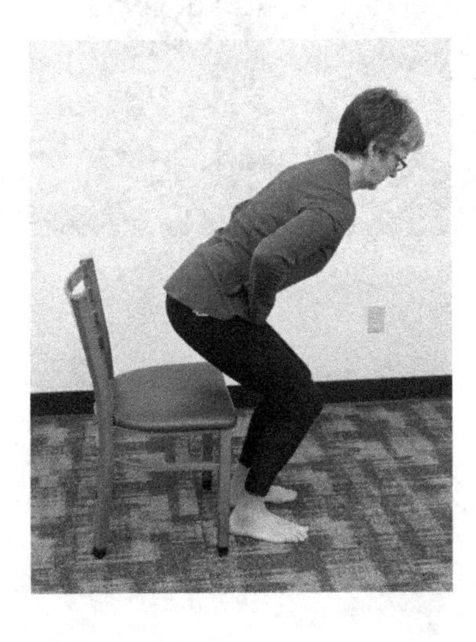

All-Fours Leg Lift

- Position yourself on your hands and knees with your head, cage, and pelvis lined up in neutral, which requires directing your gaze to the ground. There should be a low-grade tension (level 1) throughout the Encasement muscle to hold the belly in this position. Avoid giving in to the sag.
- Initiate the movement of lifting one leg with an exhale and ratcheting up tension of the Encasement to level 2. Revert to tension level 1 when the leg has returned to start position.
- Progress this exercise by repeatedly lifting and extending the leg for 30 repetitions before returning to start position.
- For an additional challenge, simultaneously lift and reach out with the opposite arm as you lift the leg.

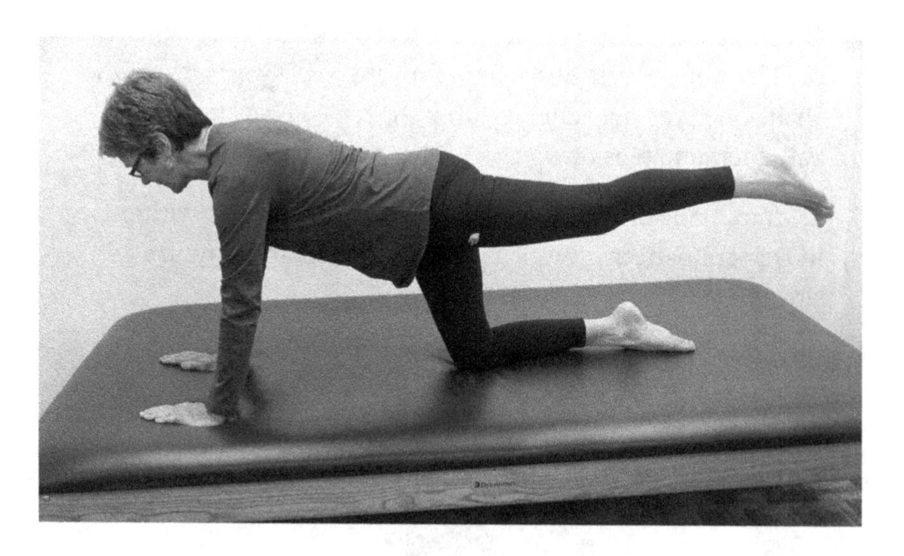

Single Leg Balance with Side Kick

- Begin in a neutral standing posture with your weight evenly distributed on both feet and holding a tension level 1.
- Increase the tension level to 2 as you shift your weight to one foot and bring the other foot off the ground, maintaining a straight knee
- Hold this position standing on one leg while you actively side kick the unloaded leg, taking care to lead with your heel.
- This exercise can be progressed with a resistance band.

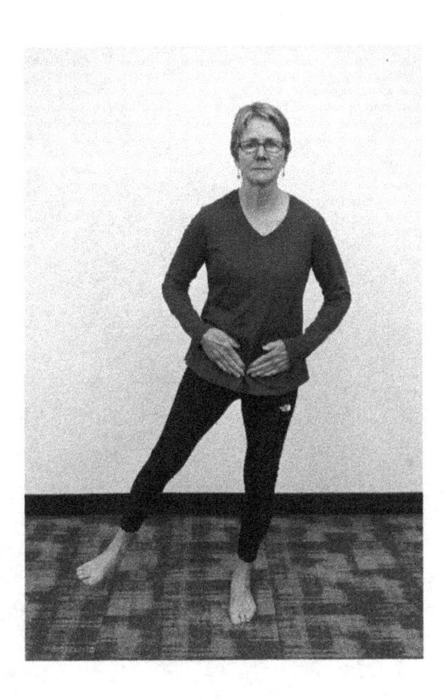

CHAPTER 17

Integrating the Core

Hopefully by now, you have a thorough awareness of how you are breathing and a newfound capability for generating the right kind of tension support for your power base. If you have any difficulty with any of the exercises previously described, then you should reach out for help. If you're having more trouble with pain, continence, or breathlessness, then you should contact a physical therapist. Talk to your trainer, a nurse practitioner, a physician, a physician assistant, or a chiropractor—anyone who is qualified to analyze your situation or knows someone who is.

It is hard to develop new muscle memories. The challenge in restoring the Inner Core is not the actual exercises or the drills. It is taking the time to build the memories. Creating or restoring a muscle memory requires dedication and an investment of time. It takes at least two weeks of practice for the memory to encode in the brain. Once the muscle activation is set, then it takes practice mixing up the intensity and duration for the activation to occur without having to think about it each time.

It is the same with posture. Almost everybody struggles with posture. Posture is just another muscle habit. If you are struggling with posture or if posture is too painful to hold, then there is a muscle that is either overworking or underworking. Usually, it's a combination of both. The overworking muscles compensate for the underworking ones. This is why bullying or forcing things is not a solution. You will only end up with more pain or more problems or both.

The challenge at this stage of the game is to hold on to what you and your body have learned so far. The final stage of owning new habits is putting them to the test with the stress of load and speed.

This chapter will present a way to safely start working toward those proverbial "Top Twenty Core Exercises" we talked about at the start of the book. Key positions and movement challenges are the basis for a variety of core exercises. When you have mastered the position movement, then you are on your way to a full core training routine that is safe and effective for improving how your body works and what you will be capable of doing.

Sit Lowering

- Sit on the ground with both legs bent at a 45-degree angle and your thorax stacked over your pelvis. Place one hand over your chest bone and the other hand over your lower belly. Your hands will help you maintain awareness of the alignment of your thorax over the pelvis, as well as of your tension support of the Encasement muscle.

- Take a deep breath in, and as you slowly exhale, extend your body from its neutral point backward to a 60-degree angle. The pivot point is your pelvis. You are literally holding the alignment of cage over pelvis while the pelvis rocks back.

- *It is important that the Encasement tension jumps up to a level 2 or higher to hold the support required to keep the thorax perfectly aligned over the pelvis at that angle.*

- Hold that position for 2 full breaths, then return to neutral. The goal is to be able to hold that position for up to 15 breaths.

- You can progress the challenge of this exercise by holding weights in your hands while doing the exercise. When this becomes easier, you can begin performing a modified press with the weights in this position.

Double Knee Lift

- Position yourself comfortably on your back with your knees bent at a 45-degree angle and your hands resting on your lower belly. Inhale and then initiate lifting one foot off the floor with the start of your exhale. Hold this position. The tension of the Encasement should be around level 2.
- *Breathe and monitor your Encasement tension with your hands. Any loss of tension will be revealed as a doming or pooch of the belly.*
- Initiate lifting the second leg to join the first one with an exhale. Hold this position, breathe, and monitor tension, holding at level 2 (though it might feel like level 3).
- Return to the start position one leg at a time.
- You can progress this exercise by extending one leg from the double-knees-up position.

Note: Both of the previous exercises are excellent for mastering the ability to do core training activities that involve crunches, Vs, and leg lifts.

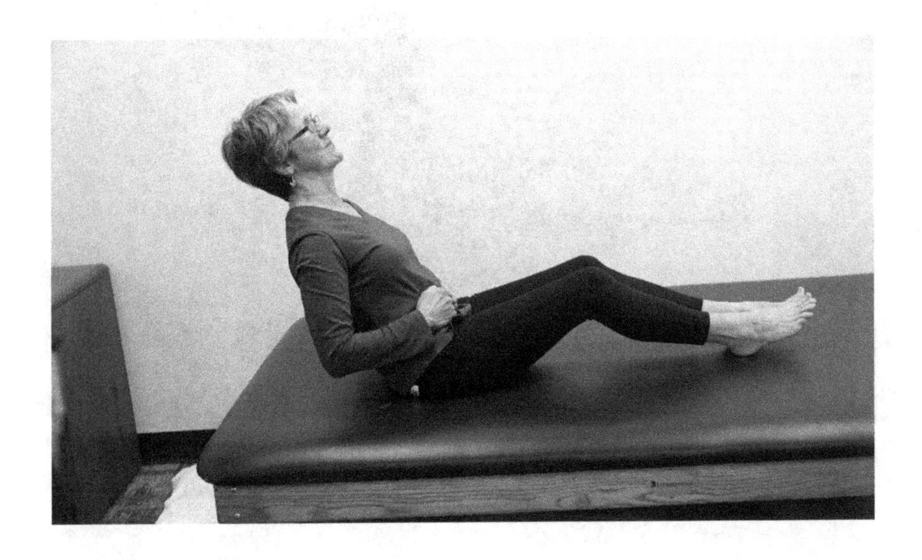

Plank

- Lie on the ground on your stomach with hands positioned under shoulders and braced. Initiate pushing into a modified plank position from the knees with an exhale and a tension level 2 of the Encasement.
- Hold the modified plank position for 2 full breath cycles before returning to the ground.
- Progress this by holding the modified plank for 15 breath cycles.
- Once this becomes natural and easy, progress to a full plank from the toes.

The plank is a platform position from which a lot of exercises work. Multiple poses in yoga, for example, move in and out of the plank, as do Pilates exercises. No "Top Twenty" core program is complete without at least three variations of using the plank. It is an incredibly hard pose to work correctly and a huge contributor to compensatory breath holding.

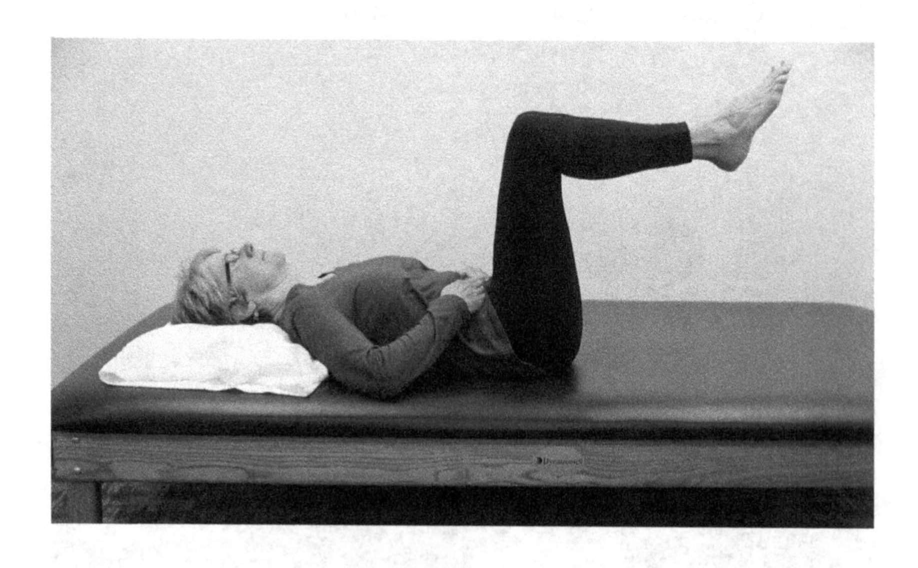

Squat

- Position yourself in standing with feet spaced shoulder width apart and weight equally distributed. A good squat requires a solid hip hinge.
- Initiate squatting down with an exhale. The primary pivot point of a squat is at the hips, leading with your tailbone, and the lesser pivot point is the knees. Keep your cage lined up over the pelvis as the body pivots.
- *Tension of the Encasement should jump up immediately to level 2 as you initiate the pivot—maybe even to level 3 if you have weights in your hands.*
- Inhale to return to standing.

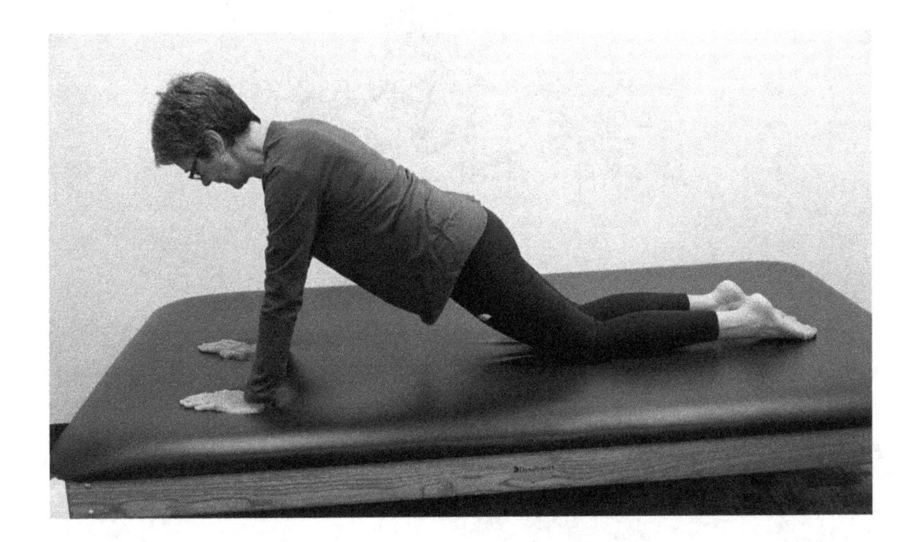

This exercise should begin with very light weights to establish the habit and pattern of how you use your breath while squatting, as well as your posture and your Encasement and Floor tensions. Moving to heavier weights may call for a different pattern. This is where you would benefit from consulting with a therapist, a fitness specialist, or a trainer who understands the mechanics of the Inner Core.

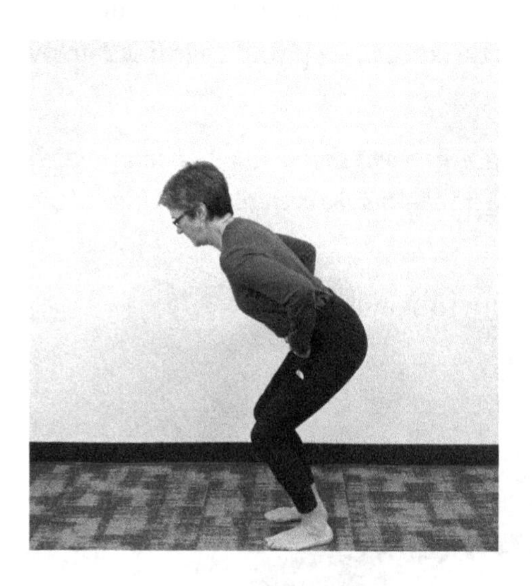

Lunge

There are multiple ways to work a lunge, which is an extremely important exercise. It is this movement that will always help you get up off the ground, even when you're eighty-five!

It's also easy to cheat with this exercise. I like to teach my clients to begin at the point of greatest challenge for them and go forward from there.

The start position requires a block (I usually use a yoga block, but any safe prop will do).

- Position yourself in a half-kneeling position with the block under the knee that is on the ground.
- Brace the toes and position the front foot under the front knee.

- *Encasement tension in this position should be around level 1 (though it may feel like level 2 for some).*
- Initiate the movement with an exhale and ramp up the tension by one degree as you shift your weight forward onto the front leg.
- Lift the body up and hold at the point where the knee clears the block.
- Hold that position for 2 breaths.
- Progress this exercise by holding the lift up to 15 breaths.
- Be sure to do both legs!

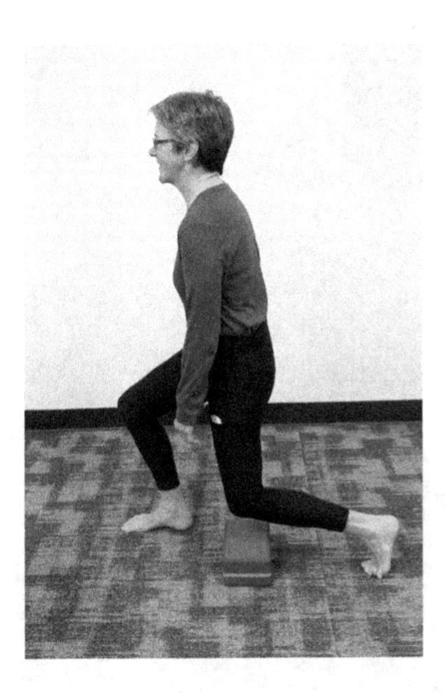

CONCLUSION

Core Grace for Moving Forward

Grace is defined by beautiful movement. It is a pleasure to watch people move well in their bodies. Moving well has nothing to do with the amount of weight a body is carrying nor where the weight is carried within the body. It has to do with how we use our muscles to hold our body. Posture and movement reflect strength, character, and capability. The more effective you are with your muscle control, the more effective you are in your body, and it shows in how you move.

People watching is a favorite pastime for those of us who make our living in the business of physical therapy. Therapists have invested a significant amount of time studying what movement can tell us about a patient's pain. Movement also tells us which anatomical structures are not doing their part in the body and what structures are compensating for them. Watching people move well in their bodies is fascinating to me because it's all about how they control their core muscles.

By now, you have learned a lot about your core anatomy and you have gone through a self-assessment. Hopefully, you have better awareness of how you are using your core muscles. It can be very difficult to be objective about what your body is doing. After all, each muscle memory you have is what your brain has perceived as normal movement for a long time. This is particularly true for all three of the Inner Core muscles. Here are reasons to seek a therapist's help:

- If you still have questions about how you are using your Inner and Outer Core muscles, then the best option is to find a physical therapist or a good physical trainer. Although there is a lot of information on the internet, it's easy to get led astray there. Plus, it's really helpful for a more objective person to assess what you are doing. Finding a good therapist or trainer is where the internet can actually come in handy. When people ask me to help them find a therapist in another state or city, I do a search for clinics that have "manual therapy" therapists. Then I look at each one of the bios, which is where you'll find a list of the courses and training the therapists have attended. If they have a lot of training, consistently updated, from respected institutions, it may be worth scheduling an appointment.

- If you are convinced that you know how to breathe well and can engage your Encasement and your Floor, but you can't seem to get it together with integrating the exercises, then it's time to find a good trainer or therapist. There's likely a piece of coordinative training that you need to bridge that muscle integration, and a good trainer or therapist will be able to help you.
- If you start to experience pain in any part of your body that was not there prior to beginning these activities, then stop and make an appointment with a physician and a physical therapist. It might just be coincidental; however, it is wise not to make assumptions. Many times, there are old problems that wake up when we start moving. The good news is that you will be better for it. You will resolve whatever old issue is limiting you and move forward with restoring your body.
- If you are convinced that you can breathe well and can appropriately engage your Floor and Encasement while you are doing all of the transition exercises, but you are wondering how far you should go, it would be appropriate to find a good trainer and focus on moving into more challenging exercises. Having some supervision will keep your technique on board and not allow you to regress into any

old bad habits. It is not necessary to meet with a trainer every time you do your exercises, but it's a good idea to have your technique checked out every other week.

Your Time Is Valuable and So Are You!

One of the main frustrations I have observed in women doing core training is making the time for it in their busy lives. Training requires a lot of consistent practice with awareness. Research shows that regular practice as prescribed by therapists on a daily basis will make a difference in muscle memory by two weeks. Muscle memory needs to progress to the next level and be built upon in order to get the desired changes in the body's abilities. That's a lot of practice over the span of several months.

It's frustrating because something always comes up to interrupt our progress. We've all been there. Everybody falls off their practice when they go on vacation, for instance. And it's so hard to get back in the groove once you return. It's like a vacation requires a vacation to recover from being on vacation! But the point is, you'll always encounter situations and circumstances that threaten to derail your practice, especially if you have children. So it's extremely important to keep your eye on the prize. A stable, steady core training program is an investment that will undoubtedly pay off . . . but there is a process to follow.

An issue that regularly arises here in Alaska, where I live, entails work activity that requires more exertion than your body is used to. Particularly during the fishing season, when the salmon are running, everybody is working harder and longer than usual. That means soreness and stiffness. Anytime pain enters the picture, there's the tendency to fall back into old muscle memory patterns. This also happens when we get tired. Muscle fatigue virtually always results in falling back on what the brain and body know best.

Whether you're detoured by life events, pain, fatigue, or all of the above, you can reset, recover, and move forward. Many people get aggravated by all the interruptions to their new routine and just give up. It's easy to believe that the work you did was all for naught, but that's not the case. The reality is that it takes time to grow both your body's capacity and your brain's coordination capabilities. When you can dedicate the time, you'll get the results.

Successful Aging

The term "successful aging" is a way of describing the quality of life you will have as you get older. Aging is very frightening to many people because it just seems to be a process of losing control of your body and your life. There is also a lot of pain associated with this process. Though it's true that our bodies do change as we get older, it is possible to prepare for those changes and meet them effectively.

How your physical body is working plays a huge role in how well you are living life. Most of us want to hold on to all our senses, and the ability to move well is a big part of this. So many social and intellectual activities are easier to participate in when we can freely use our physical bodies. Adapting to change and staying actively engaged are major themes in successful aging.

Many women seem to believe that their bodies will just stop working at some point and there's nothing to be done about that. This is simply not true. If you have a functioning nervous system attached to a physical body, then you can change it and improve how you feel and how you move.

Recover Your Core Grace

About five years ago, I was at a Cirque du Soleil show watching the incredible control of the dancers. Their core muscle control was amazing. What struck me the most was the ease and coordination built into every movement and maneuver. None of the dancers had massive shoulder muscles or ripped abs. Despite the apparent lack of muscle mass, these dancers had the ability to support their bodies in a full lateral plank with just their arms holding on to a pole like a flag. This proves that you don't need huge muscles generating lots of power to restore beautiful movement and grace. That's the job of coordination and muscle control. The ultimate control involves harnessing the power of breath and using every possible tension point at the right amount and at the right time.

Everyone can recover this kind of control and movement. No matter your age or your shape, it is possible to recover. The key is a combination of practice, awareness, and building movement activity into your life. This means regular walks, exercise classes that you enjoy, bowling with friends. Whatever brings you pleasure will benefit you if it involves regular activity. So stay mobile, tend to your core, and make the most of your life.

References

Almeida V, Guimaraes F, Moco V, et al. Is there an association between postural balance and pulmonary function in adults with asthma? *Clinics*. 2013; 68(11): 1421–1427.

Almousa S, Loon A. The prevalence of urinary incontinence in nulliparous female sportswomen: A systematic review. *Journal of Sport Sciences*. 2019; 37(14): 1663–1672.

Anderson B, Bliven K. The use of breathing exercises in the treatment of chronic, non-specific low back pain. *Journal of Sports Rehabilitation*. 2017; 26: 452–458.

Arab A, Behbahani R, Lorestani L, et al. Assessment of pelvic floor function in women with and without low back pain using transabdominal ultrasound. *Manual Therapy*. 2010; 15: 235–239.

Araujo M, Brito L, Rossi F, et al. Prevalence of female urinary incontinence in crossfit practitioners and associated factors: An internet population based survey. *Female Pelvic Medicine and Reconstructive Surgery*. 2020; 26: 97–100.

Ashton-Miller J, DeLancey J. On the biomechanics of vaginal birth and common sequelae. *Annual Review of Biomedical Engineering*. 2009; 11: 163–76.

Azambuja A, Sbruzzi L. Inspiratory muscle training in patients with heart failure: What is new? Systematic review and meta-analysis. *Physical Therapy*. 2020 Sep.

Baessler K, Schmid C, Maher C, et al. Surgery for women with pelvic organ prolapse with or without stress urinary incontinence. *Cochrane Database of Systematic Reviews*. 2018; 8. CD013108.

Bains K, Kashyap S, Lappin S. StatPearls Anatomy, thorax, diaphragm. [Internet] *StatPearls Publishing*; Island (Fl); Aug 15, 2020. PMID 30137842.

Barba E, Burri E, Accarino A, et al. Abdominothoracic mechanisms of functional abdominal distension and correction by biofeedback. *Gastroenterology*. 2015; 148: 732–739.

Baruaa A, Pattnaik M, Mohanty P. Comparison of lung function of normal and persons with chronic low back pain and its relation with duration and severity of chronic low back pain. *Journal of Novel Physiotherapy and Rehabilitation*. 2017; 1: 137–143.

Beeckman N, Vermeersch A, Lysen R, et al. The presence of respiratory disorders in individuals with low back pain: A systematic review. *Manual Therapy*. 2016; 26: 77–86.

Benjamin D, van de Water A, Peiris C. Effects of exercise on diastasis of the rectus abdominis muscle in the antenatal and postnatal periods: A systematic review. *Physiotherapy*. 2014; 100: 1–8.

Bing M, Gimbel H, Greisen S, et al. Clinical risk factors and urodynamic predictors prior to surgical treatment for stress urinary incontinence: A narrative review. *International Urogynecology Journal.* 2015; 26: 175–185.

Bivia-Roig G, Lison J, Sanchez-Zuriaga. Changes in trunk posture and muscle responses in standing during pregnancy and postpartum. *PLoS One.* 13(3): e0194853.

Brech G, Plapler P, Meirelles E, et al. Evaluation of the association between osteoporosis and postural balance in postmenopausal women. *Gait and Posture.* 2013; 38: 321–325.

Briggs A, Greig A, Wark J. The vertebral fracture cascade in osteoporosis: A review of aetiopathogenesis. *Osteoporos International.* 2007; 18: 575–584.

Briggs A, Greig A, Bennell K, Hodges P. Paraspinal muscle control in people with osteoporotic vertebral fracture. *European Spine Journal.* 2007; 16 1137–1144.

Briggs A, Wrigley T, van Dieen J, et al. The effect of osteoporotic vertebral fracture on predicted spinal loads in vivo. *European Spine Journal.* 2006; 15: 1785–1795.

Broy S. The vertebral fracture cascade: Etiology and clinical implications. *Journal of Clinical Densitometry.* 2016; 19(1): 29–34.

Brumagne S, Diers M, Danneels L, et al. Neuroplasticity of sensorimotor control in low back pain. *Journal of Orthopaedic Sports Physical Therapy.* 2019; 49(6): 402–414.

Bordoni B, Morabito B, Simonelli M. Ageing of the diaphragm muscle. *Cureus.* 2020 Jan; 12(1): e6645. DOI: 10.7759/cureus.6645.

Bordoni B, Morabito B. Symptomatology correlations between the diaphragm and irritable bowel syndrome. *Cureus.* 2018; 10(7): e3036.

Borujeni B, Yalfani A. Reduction of postural sway in athletes with chronic low back pain through eight weeks of inspiratory muscle training: A randomized controlled trial. *Clinical Biomechanics.* 2019; 69: 215–220.

Bosnes I, Nordahl H, Stordal E, et al. Lifestyle predictors of successful aging: A 20 year prospective HUNT study. *PLoS One.* 14(7): e0219200.

Burri E, Barba E, Huaman J, et al. Mechanisms of postprandial abdominal bloating and dissension in functional dyspepsia. *Gut.* 2013; 63: 395–400.

Casagrande D, Gugala Z, Clark S, et al. Low back pain and pelvic girdle pain in pregnancy. *Journal of the American Academy of Orthopaedic Surgeons.* 2015 Sep; 23(9): 539–549.

Chaitow L, Bradley D, Gilbert C. *Recognizing and Treating Breathing Disorders: A Multidisciplinary Approach, 2nd ed.* Churchill Livingstone, Elsevier. 2014.

Chapman E, Hansen-Honeycutt J, May J. A clinical guide to the assessment and treatment of breathing pattern disorders in the physically active: Part 1. *International Journal of Sports Physical Therapy.* 2016 Oct; 11(5): 803–809.

Chen C, Gong X, Yang X, et al. The roles of estrogen and strogen receptors in gastrointestinal disease (Review). *Oncology Letters.* 2019; 18: 5673–5680.

Christiansen B, Bouxsein M. Biomechanics of vertebral fractures and the vertebral fracture cascade. *Current Osteoporosis Reports.* 2010; 8: 198–204.

Courtney R, Van Dixhoorn J, Cohen M. Evaluation of breathing pattern: Comparison of a Manual Assessment of Respiratory Motion (MARM) and respiratory induction plethysmography. *Applied Psychophysiology and Biofeedback.* 2008; 33: 91–100.

Craft B, Carroll H, Lustyk M. Gender differences in exercise habits and quality of life reports: Assessing the moderating effects of reasons for exercise. *International Journal of Liberal Arts and Social Science.* 2014; 2(5): 675–76.

Crossfit Games. Do You Pee During Workouts? (video). YouTube. https://youtu.be/UKzq1upNIgU. Published June 16, 2013. Accessed May 9, 2020.

Dulger E, Bilgin S, Bulut E, et al. The effect of stabilization exercises on diaphragm muscle thickness and movement in women with low back pain. *Journal of Back and Musculoskeletal Rehabilitation*. 2018; 31: 323–329.

Dumoulin C, Hunter K, Moore K, et al. Conservative management for female urinary incontinence and pelvic organ prolapse review 2013: Summary of the 5th international consultation on incontinence. *Neurology and Urodynamics*. 2016; 35: 15–20.

ElDeeb A, Hamada H, Abdel-Aziem A, et al. The relationship between trunk and pelvis kinematics during pregnancy trimesters. *Acta of Bioengineering and Biomechanics*. 2016; 18(4): 79–85.

Elks W, Jaramillo-Huff A, Barnes L, et al. The stress urinary incontinence in crossfit (SUCCeSS) study. *Female Pelvic Medicine and Reconstructive Surgery*. 2020; 26: 101–106.

Estebsari F, Dastoorpoor M, Khalifehkandi, et al. The concept of successful aging: A review article. *Current Aging Science*. 2020; 13: 4–10.

Fahmi S, Simonis F, Abayazid M. Respiratory motion estimation of the liver with abdominal motion as a surrogate. *International Journal of Medical Robotics and Computer Assisted Surgery*. 2018; 14: e1940.

Fernandes da Mota, P, Pascoal A, Carita P, et al. Prevalence and risk factors of diastasis recti abdominis from later pregnancy to 6 months postpartum, and relationship with lumbo-pelvic pain. *Manual Therapy*. 2015; 20: 200–205.

Finta R, Nagy E, Bender T. The effect of diaphragm training on lumbar stabilizer muscles: A new concept for improving segmental stability in the case of low back pain. *Dove Medical Press Limited*. 2018 Nov; 2018(11): 3031–3045.

Frank C, Kobesova A, Kolar P. Dynamic neuromuscular stabilization and sports rehabilitation. *International Journal of Sports Physical Therapy*. 2013 Feb; 8(1): 62–73.

Fritel X, Ringa V, Quiboeuf E, et al. Female urinary incontinence, from pregnancy to menopause: A review of epidemiological and pathophysiological findings. *Acta Obstetricia et Gynecologica Scandinavica*. 2012; 91: 901–910.

Fuseini H, Newcomb D. Mechanicsms driving gender differences in asthma. *Current Allergy and Asthma Reports*. 2017; 17(3): 19. DOI: 10.1007/s11882-017-0686-1.

Gilleard W, Brown JM. Structure and function of the abdominal muscles in primigravid subjects during pregnancy and the immediate postbirth period. *Physical Therapy*. 1996 Jul; 76(7): 750–762.

Goncalves M, Francisco D, deMedeiros C, et al. Postural alignment of patients with Chronic Obstructive Pulmonary Disease. *Fisioterapia Movimento*. 2017; 30(3): 549–558.

Goossens N, Rummens S, Janssens L, et al. Association between sensorimotor impairments and functional brain changes in patients with low back pain: A critical review. *American Journal of Physical Medicine and Rehabilitation*. 2018; 97(3): 200–211.

Greig A, Bennell K, Briggs A, et al. Balance impairment is related to vertebral fracture rather than thoracic kyphosis in individuals with osteoporosis. *Osteoporosis International*. 2007; 18: 543–551.

Greig A, Briggs A, Bennell K, Hodges P. Trunk muscle activity is modified in osteoporotic vertebral fracture and thoracic kyphosis with potential consequences for vertebral health. *PLoS One*. 2014; 9(10): e109515.

Hagin M, Pietrek M, Sheikhzadeh A, et al. The effects of breath control on intra-abdominal pressure during lifting tasks. *Spine.* 2004; 29(4); 464–469.

Hodges P, Cholewicki J. Functional Control of the Spine. In: Vleeming A, Mooney V, Stoeckart R. *Movement, Stability, and Lumbopelvic Pain.* Churchill Livingstone: Elsevier; 2007: 489–512.

Hodges P, Danneels L. Changes in structure and function of the back muscles in low back pain: Different time points, observations, and mechanisms. *Journal of Orthopaedic and Sports Physical Therapy.* 2019; 49(6): 464–476.

Hodges P, Ferreira P, Ferreira M. Lumbar Spine: Treatment of Motor Control Disorders. In: Magee D, Zachazewski J, Quillen W, Manske R. *Pathology and Intervention in Musculoskeletal Rehabilitation, 2nd ed.* Maryland Heights, Missouri: Elsevier; 2016: 520–560.

Hodges P, Mosely GL, Gabrielsson A, et al. Experimental muscle pain changes feedforward postural responses of the trunk muscles. *Exp Brain Res.* 2003; 151: 262–271.

Iqbal M, Hussain T, Khalid F, et al. Diastasis Recti Abdominis and its associated risk factors in postpartum women. *Pak Armed Forces Med J.* 2020; 70(5): 1535–38.

Janssens L, Brumagne S, McConnell A, et al. Proprioceptive changes impair balance control in individuals with Chronic Obstructive Pulmonary Disease. *PLoS One.* 2013 Mar; 8(3): e57949.

Janssens L, McConnell A, Pijnenburg M, et al. Inspiratory muscle training affects proprioceptive use and low back pain. *Medicine and Science in Sports and Exercise.* 2014. DOI: 10.1249/MSS.0000000000000385.

Kanis J, McCloskey E, Harvey N, et al. Intervention thresholds and the diagnosis of osteoporosis. *Journal of Bone and Mineral.* 2015 Oct; 30(10): 1747–1753.

Kelley G, Kelley K, Kohrt W. Effects of ground and joint reaction force exercise on lumbar spine and femoral neck bone mineral density in postmenopausal women: A meta analysis of randomized controlled trials. *BMC Musculoskeletal Disorders.* 2012; 13: 177.

Kera T, Maruyama H. The effects of posture on respiratory activity of abdominal muscles. *Journal of Physiological Anthropology and Applied Human Sciences.* 2005; 24(4): 259–265.

Key J. 'The Core': Understanding it and retraining its dysfunction. *Journal of Bodywork and Movement Therapies.* 2013; 17: 541–559.

Khadgi B, Karki A, Acharya R. Does parity affect abdominal endurance causing low back pain among women. *BJHS.* 2019 Dec; 4(3) 10: 791–795.

Ki C, Heo M, Kim E. The effects of forced breathing exercise on the lumbar stabilization in chronic low back pain patients. *Journal of Physical Therapy Science.* 2016 Dec; 28(12): 3380–3383.

Kim Y, Kim N. Sex-gender differences in irritable bowel syndrome. *Journal of Neurogastoenterology and Motility.* 2018 Oct; 24(4): 544–558.

Kleim J, Jones T. Principles of experience-dependent neural plasticity: Implications for rehabilitation after brain damage. *Journal of Speech, Language, and Hearing Research.* 2008 Feb; 51: S225–S239.

Kocjan J, Adamek M, Gzik-Zroske B, et al. Network of breathing. Multifunctional role of the diaphragm. *Advances in Respiratory Medicine.* 2017; 85: 224–232.

Kocjan J, Gzik-Zroska B, Nowakowska K, et al. Impact of diaphragm function parameters on balance maintenance. *PLoS One.* 2018; 13(12): e0208697.

Kolar P, Sulc J, Kyncl M, et al. Postural function of the diaphragm in persons with and

without chronic low back pain. *Journal of Orthopedic and Sports Physical Therapy.* 2012 Apr; 42(4): 352–362.
Krkeljas Z. Changes in gait and posture as factors of dynamic stability during walking in pregnancy. *Human Movement Science.* 2018; 58: 315–320.
Lee D. *The Pelvic Girdle: An Integration of Clinical Expertise and Research, 4th ed.* Churchill Livingstone: Elsevier; 2011.
Lee D. *Diastasis Rectus Abdominis: A Clinical Guide for Those Who Are Split Down the Middle.* Surrey BC Canada: Learn with Diane Lee; 2017.
Maher C, Feiner B, Baessler K, et al. Surgical Management of pelvic organ prolapse in women. *Cochrane Database of Systematic Reviews.* 2013;4. CD004014.
Malagelada J, Accarino A, Azpiroz F. Bloating and abdominal distension: Old misconceptions and current knowledge. *American Journal of Gastroenterology.* 2017; 112: 1221–1231.
Marques E, Mota J, Machado L, et al. Multicomponent training program with weight bearing exercises elicits favorable bone density, muscle strength, and balance adaptations in older women. *Calcified Tissue International.* 2011; 88: 117–129.
Mayer E, Naliboff B, Lee O, et al. Review article: Gender-related differences in functional gastrointestinal disorders. *Alimentary Pharmacology and Therapeutics.* 1999; 13 (Suppl. 2): 65–69.
McMillan L, Zengin A, Ebeling P, et al. Prescribing physical activity for the prevention and treatment of osteoporosis in older adults. *Healthcare.* 2017; 5, 85. DOI:10.3390/healthcare5040085.
McPhee J, French D, Jackson D, et al. Physical activity in older age: Perspectives for healthy ageing and frailty. *Biogerontology.* 2016; 17: 567–580.
Mohan V, Paungmali A, Sitilerpisan P, et al. Respiratory characteristics of individuals with non-specific low back pain: A cross-sectional study. *Nursing and Health Sciences.* 2018; 20: 224–230.
Moossdorff-Steinhauser H, Berghmans B, Spaanderman M, et al. Prevalence, incidence and bothersomeness of urinary incontinence in pregnancy: A systematic review and meta-analysis. *International Urogynecology Journal.* https://doi.org/10.1007/s00192-020-04636-3.
Mota M, Cardoso M, Carvalho A, et al. Women's experience of low back pain during pregnancy. *Journal of Back and Musculoskeletal Rehabilitation.* 2015; 28: 351–357.
Nager C, Visco A, Richter H, et al. Effect of vaginal mesh hysteropexy vs vaginal hysterectomy with uterosacral ligament suspension on treatment failure in women with uterovaginal prolapse: A randomized clinical study. *JAMA.* w019; 322(11): 1054–1065.
Nawrocka A, Mynarski W, Cholewa J. Adherence to physical activity guidelines and functional fitness of elderly women using objective measurement. *Annals of Agricultural and Environmental Medicine.* 2017; 24(4): 632–635.
Nawrocka A, Niestroj-Jaworska M, Mynarski A, et al. Association between objectively measured physical activity and musculoskeletal disorders, and perceived work ability among adult middle aged and older women. *Dove Press: Clinical Intervention in Aging.* 2019; 14: 975–1983.
Nikander R, Kannus P, Dastidar P, et al. Targeted exercise against hip fragility. *Osteoporosis International.* 2009; 20: 1321–1328.
Nikander N, Sievanen H, Heinonen A, et al. Targeted exercise against osteoporosis: A

systematic review and meta-analysis for optimizing bone strength throughout life. *BMC Medicine*. 2010; 8: 47.

Olsson A, Kiwanuka O, Wilhelmsson S, et al. Cohort study of the effect of surgical repair of symptomatic diastasis recti abdominis on abdominal trunk function and quality of life. *BJS Open*. 2019 Dec; 3(6): 750–758.

Petros P, Skilling P. Pelvic floor rehabilitation in the female according to the integral theory of female urinary incontinence. *European Journal of Obstetrics and Gynecology and Reproductive Biology*. 2001; 94: 264–269.

Pisani G, Sato T, Carvalho C, et al. Impact of urinary incontinence on quality of life in female crossfit practitioners: A cross sectional study. *European Journal of Obstetrics and Gynecology and Reproductive Biology*. 2022; 268: 56–61.

Pisani G, Sato T, Carvalho C. Pelvic floor dysfunction and associated factors in female crossfit practitioners: A cross-sectional study. *International Urogynecology Journal*. 2021; 32: 2975–2984.

Ratnovsky A, Elad D, Halpern P. Mechanics of respiratory muscles. *Respiratory Physiology and Neurobiology*. 2008; 163: 82–89.

Rebullido T, Gomez- Tomas C, Faigenbaum A, et al. The prevalence of urinary incontinence among adolescent female athletes: A systematic review. *Journal of Functional Morphology and Kinesiology*. 2021; 6, 12. https://doi.org/10.3390/jfmk6010012.

Roussel N, Nijs J, Truijen S, et al. Altered breathing patterns during lumbopelvic motor control tests in chronic low back pain: A case-control study. *European Spine Journal*. 2009; 18: 1066–1073.

Sapsford R, Hodges P. Contraction of pelvic floor muscles during abdominal maneuvers. *Archives of Physical Medicine and Rehabilitation*. 2001 Aug; 82: 1081–1088.

Sapsford R, Hodges P, Richardson C, et al. Co-activation of the abdominal and pelvic floor muscles during voluntary exercises. *Neurourology and Urodynamics*. 2001; 20: 31–42.

Sherburn M, Guthrie J, Dudley E, et al. Is incontinence associated with menopause? *Obstetrics and Gynecology*. 2001; 98(4): 628–633.

Sjodahl J, Kvist J, Gutke A, et al. A methodological electromyography study in parous women without lumbopelvic pain. *Clinical Biomechanics*. 2009; 24: 183–189.

Smith M, Chang A, Hodges P. Balance recovery is compromised and trunk muscle activity is increased in chronic obstructive pulmonary disease. *Gait and Posture*. 2016; 43: 101–107.

Smith M, Russell A, Hodges P. Disorders of breathing and continence have a stronger association with back pain than obesity and physical activity. *Australian Journal of Physiotherapy*. 2006; 52: 11–16.

Smith M, Russell A, Hodges P. The relationship between incontinence, breathing disorders, gastrointestinal symptoms, and back pain in women: a longitudinal study. *The Clinical Journal of Pain*. 2014; 30(2): 162–167.

Sperstad J, Tennfijord M, Hilde G, et al. Diastasis recti abdominis during pregnancy and 12 months after childbirth: Prevalence, risk factors, and report of lumbopelvic pain. *British Journal of Sports Medicine*. 2016; 50: 1092–1096.

Sullivan S. Functional abdominal bloating with distension. *ISRN Gastroenterology*. 2012. DOI:10.5402/2012/721820.

Szczgiel E, Blaut J, Zielonka-Pycka K, et al. The impact of deep muscle training on the quality of posture and breathing. *Journal of Motor Behavior*. 2018; 50(2); 219–227.

Talasz H, Kremser C, Kofler M, et al. Phase locked parallel movement of diaphragm

and pelvic floor during breathing and coughing: A dynamic MRI investigation in healthy females. *International Urogynecology Journal*. 2011; 22: 61–68.
Talasz H, Kremser C, Kofler M, et al. Proof of concept: Differential effects of Valsalva and straining maneuvers on the pelvic floor. *European Journal of Obstetrics and Gynecological and Reproductive Biology*. 2012; 164: 227–233.
Teymuri Z, Hosseinifar M, Sirousi M. The effect of stabilization exercises on pain, disability, and pelvic floor muscle function in postpartum lumbopelvic pain. *American Journal of Physical Medicine and Rehabilitation*. 2018; 97: 885–891.
Thomas M, McKinley R, Freeman E, et al. Breathing retraining for dysfunctional breathing in asthma: A randomized controlled trial. *Thorax*. 2003; 58: 110–115.
Troy K, Mancuso M, Butler T, et al. Exercise early and often: Effects of physical activity and exercise on women's bone health. *International Journal of Environmental Research and Public Health*. 2018; 15. DOI: 10.3390/ijerph15050878.
Trueland J. Childbirth, menopause, ageing, and stress incontinence: Dispelling the myths. *Nursingstandard.com*. 2020 Sep; 35(9): 51–53.
Urquhart D, Hodges P, Story I. Postural activity of the abdominal muscles varies between regions of these muscles and between body positions. *Gait and Posture*. 2005; 22: 295–301.
Van Dieen J, Reeves P, Kawchuk G, et al. Analysis of motor control in patients with low back pain: A key to personalized care? *Journal of Orthopaedic and Sports Physical Therapy*. 2019; 49(6): 380–388.
Vikhe B, Bhalerao M. Study of forced expiratory volume in one second and forced vital capacity in normal pregnancy from Western Maharashtra. *National Journal of Physiology, Pharmacy and Pharmacology*. 2019; 9(11): 1130–1133.
Villoria A, Azpiroz F, Burri E, et al. Abdomino-phrenic dyssynergia in patients with abdominal bloating and distension. *American Journal of Gastroenterology*. 2011; 106: 815–819.
Vostatek P, Novak D, Rychnovsky T, et al. Diaphragm postural function analysis using magnetic resonance imaging. *PLoS One*. 2013; 8(3): e56724.
Wales K, Gray T. Urinary incontinence in women. *InnovAiT*. 2019; 12(12): 690–696.
Wallace S, Miller L, Mishra K. Pelvic floor physical therapy in the treatment of pelvic floor dysfunction in women. *Current Opinion in Gynecology*. 2019; 31(6): 485–493.
Weintraub A, Glinter H, Marcus-Baun N. Narrative review of the epidemiology, diagnosis, and pathophysiology of pelvic organ prolapse. *International Brazilian Journal of Urology*. 2020; 46: 5–14.
Wikander L, Kirshbaum M, Gahreman D. Urinary incontinence and women crossfit competitors. *International Journal of Women's Health*. 2020; 12: 1189–1195.
Zein J, Erzurum S. Asthma is different in women. *Current Allergy and Asthma Reports*. 2015; 15(6): 28. DOI: 10.1007/s11882-015-0528-y.

CPSIA information can be obtained
at www.ICGtesting.com
Printed in the USA
BVHW090947270922
648083BV00008B/1016